THE
SOVEREIGN
HEALTH
SOLUTION

DR. EVA DETKO

ISBN: 978-19-5-315363-0

Published by

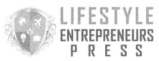

If you are interested in publishing through Lifestyle Entrepreneurs Press, write to: *Publishing@LifestyleEntrepreneursPress.com*

Publications or foreign rights acquisition of our catalog books. Learn More: *www.LifestyleEntrepreneursPress.com*

Printed in the USA

50% OFF

Dr. Eva's ADDRESSING PSYCHOENERGETIC ROOT
CAUSES OF CHRONIC ILLNESS Online Program
with this coupon code:

SOVEREIGNHEALTH2022

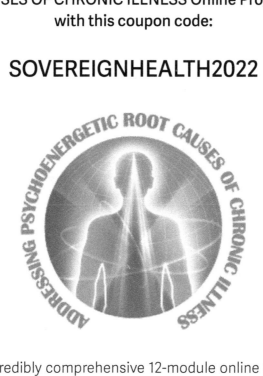

This incredibly comprehensive 12-module online program
is an extension of the book with over 90 hours of video and
audio content, guiding you step-by-step through all the key
aspects of psycho-energetic healing. The program is focused
on healing your amygdala, as well as rebalancing your nervous system and your biofield, using neuroscience-based
tools. With this in-depth practical approach you will build
neurological, emotional and energetic resilience that will
transform your mental and physical health!

To take advantage of this amazing offer go to:
www.dr-eva.com/psychoenergetic-root-causes-program

Contents

Foreword

Although we are surrounded by more technical advances than ever, the most powerful health protocols addressing almost every kind of health condition, and we can literally see into your body's cells, all the way down to your DNA, none of this matters if you do not ALSO conquer the psycho-energetic root causes of illness.

From understanding emotional toxicity and trauma, to building neurological resilience and balancing your biofield, Dr. Eva Detko's newest book explores the step-by-step process of seeing beyond symptomology and endless health hurdles and looking at the core causality that may actually live deep in the subconscious.

While modern medicine offers so many healing opportunities, it is very limited when we move beyond the realm of physical health - especially when it comes to chronic health conditions. Indeed, even limiting belief systems can completely block recovery on every level - and remain an undiagnosed, unseen villain in your health journey.

Dr. Eva Detko is a powerful healer, who goes far beyond the disease and symptom roller coaster and elevates her reader out of the billion-dollar pharmaceutical and medical industry to a place where they can create true ownership and experience sovereignty, teaching a blueprint for self-directed health and well being on every level.

As a Naturopathic Doctor, I have seen thousands of patients, who have sometimes struggled for decades and invested hundreds of thousands of dollars, only to discover that their solution lies beyond the physical - it lays deep within self-care, self-knowledge and a way of life that engages emotional and psycho-energetic solutions to support the whole person - body, mind and soul.

This book leads the reader, in a powerful, interesting and organized way through a methodology that Dr. Eva developed over two and a half decades of study and clinical practice, and incorporates the newest therapeutic modalities and techniques available, all of which can be self-directed and self-applied. Psycho-energetics is the frontier of new medicine - and this book is a powerful entrypoint to create personal agency over your well-being, armed with new tools.

Many people have limited success when trying to address their psycho-energetic health because their approach lacks direction and coherence. THIS book is filled with support, such as video education and downloadable tools, to make this opportunity realistic and employable.

At its deepest level, disease starts when we experience an energetic imbalance, blocking the energy flow in the body - and that imbalance can have physical, emotional, mental or spiritual roots. The modalities and solutions explored in this book are a roadmap to defining a totally new experience with health.

Christine Schaffner, ND
www.DrChristineSchaffner.com

THE TRIANGLE OF HEALING

YOU HAVE MORE CONTROL OVER YOUR HEALTH THAN YOU REALIZE

CREATING YOUR REALITY WITH AFFIRMATIONS & IMAGERY

RESILIENCE & THE NERVOUS SYSTEM BALANCE

SELF-AWARENESS AS THE MAIN KEY TO YOUR SUCCESS

UNDERSTANDING & MASTERING EMOTIONS

HEALING EMOTIONAL TRAUMA

ATTACHMENT TRAUMA & INNER FAMILY WORK

VALUES, BELIEFS & OPTIMIZING YOUR PROGRAMS

HEALTHY BOUNDARIES & RELATIONSHIPS

ENERGETIC ASPECTS OF HEALING & BIOFIELD OPTIMIZATION

DEFINING YOUR LIFE MEANING & PURPOSE

THE PIECES OF YOUR
PSYCHO-ENERGETIC HEALTH PUZZLE

Introduction

I decided to write this book because over two decades of study and clinical practice, as well as my own experiences, have taught me that addressing our neurological, emotional, and energetic balance is critical to overcoming ill health and achieving optimal well-being. There are many different reasons why people get sick, but I have yet to meet a person with chronic health issues who has a well-balanced nervous system and energy field. That just does not happen. As we go on, I will be explaining exactly why that is, what the root causes of those imbalances are, and what we need to do to build neurological, emotional, and energetic resilience. People rarely develop health problems overnight. For most people, it starts right at the beginning of their lives. In fact, when we discuss intergenerational and ancestral trauma, you will see that more often than not, our health challenges are predetermined before we are born. I am not talking about genetics here but rather an epigenetic imprint that can go back many generations.

How It All Started for Me

I myself had a very challenging start to life. My mom had an extremely traumatic pregnancy. Her sister died at the age of sixteen from a vaccine injury, which included loss of speech and whole-body paralysis. My mother, only twenty-two and three months pregnant at the time, found it very difficult to cope with the loss and the feelings of helplessness. She was not in a good place emotionally and developed toxemia of pregnancy that resulted in my twin dying in the womb. Her consultant said to her that her mental state was directly linked to the outcome of the pregnancy. This man was clearly ahead of his time, as this was almost 50 years ago when there was practically no conversation about the mind-body connection in the West. There were no adequate tools to help people heal trauma either.

My birth was as traumatic as the pregnancy for both me and my mother. Both our lives were under serious threat, and my mom still remembers the doctors arguing about whether they should be saving her or me. Fortunately, we both survived, but as a result of all this, I was born quite weak and vulnerable. Because the other baby had died a few weeks prior to my mom going into labor, his or her little body was decomposed at birth. They could not even tell what sex the baby was. The parts of my body that had been in contact with the other baby were not healthy, and I lost all my fingernails and toenails.

Because I was born less than six months after my mom's sister passed, I was plunged into this confusing emotional mix of love, grief, and also guilt. My grandparents never forgave themselves for letting their baby be vaccinated against their better judgment. Luckily, I did get a lot of attention and love because welcoming an infant who happened to also be my mom's first child and my grandparents' first grandchild was very healing for everybody. But despite getting much affection, particularly from my grandmother, I struggled physically and emotionally through my early and teenage years.

As a small child, I was always at the doctor's. I had frequent chest infections and all sorts of other health issues, including inflamed joints. In addition, I was very shy and a bit of a pushover, and I was bullied and abused for a number of years. Among the behavioral adaptations I developed as a result of my early traumas were overachieving and perfectionism. I had control issues and was always stressed and worried about the silliest of things. Like many traumatized people, I would spend most of my waking moments ruminating on my past or being anxious about the future. For many years, I was not able to be present or enjoy my life. Fast forward a bit and in my early twenties I found myself with a massively dysregulated autonomic nervous system as a result of all the trauma and stress. As it is the case for many people, after years of trying to compensate, my body imploded and I developed ME (myalgic encephalomyelitis) and fibromyalgia, in addition to already present Hashimoto's thyroiditis.

I very quickly realized that Rockefeller doctors were only interested in pushing drugs on me and did not have the expertise to help me recover my health. In fact, they did not even believe I could. Luckily, I remained determined to find the answers and heal physically and emotionally. I tried many different natural approaches and modalities, many of which were very helpful. However, it was not until I started doing trauma, belief, and self-worth work in my mid-twenties that I started to feel a real positive shift and my nervous, immune, and endocrine systems started to rebalance.

Thanks to this work, I have fully recovered from all these life-limiting conditions. I achieved this by combing healing my nervous system, my energy field, and my biochemistry. I love sharing what I have learned over the years with others and seeing the wonderful transformations people can achieve when they have addressed the true root causes of their health issues. I am grateful every day for where I am now and for the experiences that have led me here. I consider it a privilege to have been part of many people's health journeys, and now also yours.

The Triangle of Healing

I want to begin this book by discussing the root causes of chronic health problems. First of all, regardless of whether it is gut issues, chronic fatigue, heart disease, autoimmune disease, or cancer, there is no one reason for the problem you are experiencing. This is why you have to be super cautious and run away from anyone who ever tells you that you just have to do this one thing, or take this one supplement, or eat this one food, and it will solve your problem.

My way of looking at healing is recognizing three funda-mental areas that are tightly connected and affect one another. Those three areas are:

- the physical body (includes physiological, biochemical, and mechanical factors)
- the mind (includes psychological, mental, and emo-tional factors)
- the energy field or the biofield (includes our overall ener-getic balance, as well as our spiritual connection).

Just to clarify, emotions and thoughts are energy as well, as ultimately everything is energy, but I have divided these factors in this way to help the understanding.

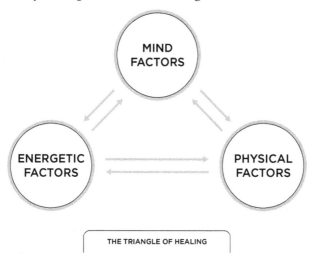

THE TRIANGLE OF HEALING

This is what I call the Triangle of Healing, in which everything affects everything else. So your thoughts and emotions affect the physical body. They affect your nervous, immune, and endocrine systems, as well as your energy field, because they are energy. Eating the wrong foods affects the body's nutritional status and it also affects neurotransmitters in the gut, which, in turn, impacts your mind and your emotional state. Foods have frequencies, and those frequencies affect the biofield. Our biofield dictates our health in every way, so if there is a disruption in our field, functioning of our cells, organs, and body systems will be impaired. Disrupted energy fields also create a higher potential for low-vibrational, dense states of consciousness like fear, anger, sadness, etc. Once you are in a chronic-disease state, it is very easy to perpetuate it because everything affects everything else. So many people find themselves on this merry-go-round. Chronic diseases are responsible for seven out of ten deaths in the U.S., so this really is a big problem.

The first thing most people do, after they have realized that conventional medicine has little to offer them for their chronic health complaints, is try to interrupt this disease cycle at the physical level. Usually, they make attempts to eat better, take supplements, and/or exercise more. Controlling the physical is the easiest in a sense because it is most tangible, and once people understand what they need to do, they either do it or they do not. It is, indeed, a great start, and many will be rewarded with some improvement in their symptoms. However, if nothing else is addressed, that result will be either short-lived, or it will take them some of the way towards their health goals and then they will plateau. This is because in the majority of cases, it is the psycho-energetic factors that are the actual root cause of ill health. It is my opinion that pretty much every single chronic health issue will have a psycho-energetic component. It is not the question of whether that piece is there but rather it is a question of how large that piece is.

Safety Is Everything

Why do I believe that? From the point of view of human nervous system development, safety is paramount. When we do not feel safe, our stress response kicks in, which, if chronic, means we cannot heal our tissues, digest our food, or detoxify. In fact, many of the body's vital processes are compromised when we spend too much time in survival states of fight, flight, or freeze. That is because the body's activities, such as digestion, detoxification, reproduction, and tissue regeneration are associated with the relaxation response (rest-digest-detoxify-healresponse), and for us to feel relaxed, we need to feel safe. We will be looking at nervous system regulation in more detail as we discuss building neurological resilience, but for now, let us focus on that safety aspect.

This is an issue for many people as early as the womb. When a pregnant woman is in distress because she is depressed, has problems at work, or worries about the finances, the impulses from her nervous system and the hormonal milieu signal to the baby that there is a threat. This is true for anything that puts the mother into survival states of fight, fight, or freeze. The nervous system responds the same whether a stressor is emotional, chemical, biological (pathogens), or mechanical.

However, it is emotional stress that tends to be there all the time for many people, due to extremely high prevalence of emotional toxicity (more about that later). That leads to the fight or flight, or even freeze, response being turned on too frequently, if not constantly. As an example, if the mother has poor self-worth and she feels unlovable, she does not just experience this some of the time. The unworthiness and self-loathing are there ALL the time. That is just one example of what comprises emotional toxicity, which is a massive contributor to nervous system dysregulation. This is obviously true for any person or child.

When we are in and out of those survival states all the time, the hormonal milieu is set for danger and the brain and the nervous system are on standby to deal with any potential threats. As a result of all this, the balance between the fight-or-flight and the rest-digest-detoxify-heal parts of the nervous system is disturbed. If that happens during pregnancy, the baby is already born wired for stress. The body adapts and learns to expect stress and wants to be prepared for it. This actually changes the brain and how the nervous system behaves. Early exposure to stress tends to set up the brain to be stuck in a vicious cycle of limbic overload (limbic kindling). This is, in turn, associated with brain inflammation and hypersensitivity to different stressors, including chemical and emotional stressors. Once trauma is encoded in the brain, particularly in the first few years of our lives, we become more susceptible to further trauma. When we become wired for stress, this also contributes to the development of different personality traits and behavioral adaptations.

In addition to a traumatic pregnancy and/or birth, the baby may not have an opportunity to bond with the mother. And what if the mother develops postnatal depression? Perhaps there are financial pressures and the mother has to go straight back to work after giving birth. Or the mother might simply not have a clue how to properly satisfy the emotional needs of the child. She is just doing the best she can, but it is vital to understand that it is the child's perspective that counts. If the child does not feel their needs are being met, that will lead to further issues. I am not even mentioning cases of actual neglect and abuse here. I hope you can now appreciate how many different factors can play a role in wiring this child for stress. As a side note, later on in the book we will also look at intergenerational trauma and its impact on our system as another critical component.

One very important thing to understand is that from birth to four years of age, we are particularly vulnerable and delicate. We are completely dependent on our caregivers. In addition, we are not able to rationalize what is going on around us because it is not until the age of 10 – 11 that our logical, rational mind develops more fully. What this means is that in the first few years of our lives, we operate predominantly in the subconscious mode. We take everything at face value and interpret the world based on how it makes us feel.

So, for example, a child may be very excited about something. They run to their parent, and the parent, who has just been looking at the bills and is extremely stressed about the finances, yells at the child: *Not now! I am busy. Leave me alone!* The child's safety is now threatened because there is yelling and, of course, their needs are not being met. They feel horrible inside. They feel rejected and unloved. But because they do not yet have the ability to understand this on the conscious level, they cannot see the parental worry or anything else that may be making the parent react in this way. All they feel is rejected. They conclude that if the parent has no time for them and yells at them, it must be their fault. It must be because they are unlovable.

Another example is when a child accidently breaks something and mother or father gets angry because they have an attachment to the item. The parent yells at a child: *Look at what you've done! How can you be so clumsy?* The child accepts that the parent is right: they are clumsy. Again, they feel useless, rejected, and unlovable. Why? Because the parent is their authority. The parent is bigger, stronger, able to communicate better, and the child simply depends on them. The authority says: *You are clumsy*; therefore, that must be true. Those first few years is when we form our core beliefs about the world and ourselves. Because even with the best of intentions, it is very easy for a small child to feel wounded inside. Unfortunately, the majority of children by the age of four will have that feeling that there is something wrong with them. That in some way *they are not OK*. That then leads to all sorts of adaptations, traumas, more limiting beliefs, and unhelpful behavioral patterns.

13

So the key point here is this: either actual or perceived lack of safety and not having our needs met when we are children has a negative impact on our developing brain and the nervous system. This coupled with other traumas and negative conditioning will contribute to the brain and nervous system becoming imbalanced and dysfunctional over time. This, in turn, impacts our hormonal balance, our microbiome, and our body's ability to digest and assimilate food, fight pathogens, control inflammation, as well as regulate blood sugar. It also impacts something called the cell danger response, which affects our mitochondrial function. When we go into this self-preservation mode as a result of trauma, this does not just happen at the psychological level. Our cells also get stuck in this red-alert state. When our mitochondria become dysfunctional, this has a knock-on effect throughout the body. The number one symptom of this is chronic fatigue.

So when you hear people talk about the gut being the root cause of all ill health, you should be asking: "Fine, but what messed up the gut in the first place?" When you look more deeply, you will soon see that the true root cause goes beyond the gut. An imbalanced nervous system that originates in childhood as a result of early exposure to stress absolutely contributes to leaky gut and poor microbiome health. Even when people say the root cause is an infection (e.g., SIBO, Candida, Epstein Barr, or Borrelia) or environmental toxicity, we have the same problem. Early exposure to stress contributes to the sympathetic branch of the nervous system firing more readily while at the same time the rest-digest-detoxify-heal response is weak and does not engage readily enough. This imbalance, if not properly addressed, becomes more pronounced over time and weakens the body's ability to defend itself against infections, or neutralize and eliminate toxins. This does not mean that omnipresent toxicity is not a problem or that once we become toxic, we should not address it. We definitely should. However, people with better neurological and energetic balance (resilience) are not as susceptible. Clearly, not everybody gets equally affected by environmental toxicity or infections, and no, we cannot just blame it on genetics (as we will discuss shortly).

Our bodies are designed to spend most of the time in the rest-digest-detoxify-heal response. People who are able to do that do not get sick. It is as simple as that. But for pretty much everybody with chronic illness, that is not the case. If you have a chronic health issue, I can pretty much guarantee that your autonomic nervous system is dysregulated, and your brain and biofield are out of balance. As I have already said, when that is the case, the body will struggle to heal, regenerate and perform many of its vital functions, including fight inflammation, which is a feature of pretty much every chronic illness.

Viewing Disease from the Energetic Perspective

Everything is energy. The human body is energy that simply slowed down enough to be solid. Our energetic health is critical to our physical health, but unfortunately, this is largely underestimated and overlooked in the West. Ultimately, health is all about resonance. From the energetic perspective, disease is simply a state of consciousness. When you spend most of your time in high states of consciousness from the point of frequency and vibration (love, joy, happiness, compassion, truth, peace), you cannot maintain a disease consciousness at the same time. Why? That high frequency will dissolve or transmute anything which is associated with low-vibrational frequencies and that includes disease. Your mind is the most powerful factor here. So if you believe you deserve to be sick, or that something will make you sick, or you are genetically predisposed to get a certain illness, you will create exactly that based on the belief that you hold and the resonance associated with that belief. On the other hand, you will have a completely different outcome if you believe you are capable of healing and are deserving of good health.

External traumatic events hold energy. You experience them as an emotion or a range of emotions. This, of course, immediately influences the physical body, including via affecting brain wave activity, activating different branches of the autonomic nervous system, and influencing secretion of hormones and neurotransmitters. This is not necessarily a problem if that emotional energy is quickly digested and discharged. However, if the emotion is too intense, you will most likely feel some of it and shut the rest of it off. That emotion then settles in the emotional body. It also moves into the mental body as you begin to create beliefs, "truths," based on that emotional experience. If not processed correctly, this energy will sooner or later move to the physical body, and that is when you may start manifesting symptoms. So the problem is not the emotional energy per sé, but rather creating resistance and attachment, which interferes with discharging that emotional energy. That is where illness and suffering ultimately stems from.

When the energy that is the emotion created by this external event is not cleared and it anchors itself in the emotional body, you will then be attracting experiences that validate that emotion and associated beliefs. For example, if somebody believes people are going to let them down or abandon them, they will tend to attract partners that will do exactly that. Somebody who believes they are a loser may, among other things, gravitate towards jobs they cannot keep. They will be attracting experiences that validate their beliefs and perpetuate them, creating yet more of that same emotional energy. This is largely subconscious. The bigger this grows, the more it is going to affect the physical body.

On the other hand, if a person allows that emotional charge to move through them, which depends on their neurological, emotional, and energetic resilience in that moment, this energy will not cause any major issues with the mental or physical body. This is why building resilience, which I will be teaching you how to do, is so critically important for preventing future trauma or minimizing its impact. In order to be able to do that, we need to comprehensively address emotional toxicity and energetic imbalances. That is what we are going to do, step by step, in this book.

Addressing All the Layers

It is important to emphasize that once the different layers of our system have been affected, we have to address that accordingly. In addition to trauma work, if the mental body is affected and the beliefs have formed, we have to deal with the beliefs. When our biology is affected and there are disruptions at the physical level, it is necessary to address the problem at that level as well as treat the root cause. Again, if a child is stewing in stress hormones and pro-inflammatory cytokines at a really young age, that will impact not just their mental and emotional health but their biology going forward. So we do need to support the body through dietary interventions to balance blood sugar and the HPA (hypothalamic-pituitary-adrenal) axis. We might also want to take some supplements to support cell membranes and mitochondria, rebalance neurotransmitters, optimize immune and brain function, or address pyroluria.

Finally, we need to consider lifestyle factors, such as circadian rhythm management, EMF protection, and moving our body. A correct assessment will help you work out what it is that you need to do at the biochemical level. These factors are important to address because the biology that is negatively impacted may hinder any work you are doing at the psycho-energetic level. However, if you are going to fully heal successfully, you need to rewire your brain and rebalance your autonomic nervous system, as well as your biofield. Just changing your diet or taking supplements will not be enough. In fact, if you have difficulties dropping into the rest-digest-detoxify-heal response easily, whatever you are doing nutritionally will be limited. That is because your ventral vagus nerve, which is the key nerve associated with the relaxation response, must be activated for your digestive and many other organs to function properly.

Who Will Benefit from the Approach Presented in This Book?

The *Sovereign Health Solution* is for:

- anyone who wants to learn about psycho-energetic aspects of healing
- anyone who may have already done some work in this area but feels like they want to address their psycho-energetic healing in a more structured way
- anyone who is feeling emotionally challenged, or who has a history of trauma
- anyone with chronic health complaints who has tried many different approaches and still isn't where they want to be.

It is very difficult to estimate how long it is going to take you to work through this method. In some ways, self-development work never ends. We can always do more work to increase our level of resilience, our connection to ourselves, or to become a better version of who we currently are. But I am talking here about doing the main chunk of your trauma, belief and self-worth work. The time this will take you depends on: whether you have done any of this work previously, the extent of what you need to address and heal, and how committed you are to the process. Most people who take my *Addressing Psycho-energetic Root Causes of Chronic Illness* online program (which is the online extension of this book) take 6 to 12 months to complete it. Some take longer, which is absolutely fine. I encourage you to view this process as an exciting road trip. Even though, you do want to keep your focus on where you are going, you also want to enjoy the journey.

What We Are Aiming to Achieve with This Approach?

By working through the method and engaging with homework, hopefully you will:

- recognize what is making you emotionally toxic and gain control of your emotional responses
- learn how to create the reality that you want
- understand how your mind and your nervous system works
- identify your secondary gain/gains
- develop deeper understanding of yourself and others
- achieve internal coherence and congruence
- heal past traumas
- prioritize values and identify value conflicts
- redesign your belief system so it actually serves you

- develop a great sense of self-worth and self-acceptance
- discover where you are on energetic sensitivity spectrum and how to set energetic boundaries
- be better connected to yourself and people you care about
- learn about different modalities that can help you balance your energy field
- learn a range of super effective techniques and tools and become proficient at managing your day-to-day stress
- make yourself neurologically, emotionally and energetically more resilient, which will have a positive impact on your mental and physical health.

My method is a culmination of almost two and a half decades of study and clinical practice, as well as my own personal experiences. It brings together many different modalities and influences: Havening Techniques®, hypnotherapy, NLP (neuro-linguistic programming), Transactional Analysis, psychoneuroimmunology, mindfulness, meditation, breath work, and a number of energy medicine modalities, including bioenergetics. By engaging actively with the method presented here, you will have a positive impact on your physical health. You might even be able to resolve your chronic issues, as many of my clients have been able to do.

When you heal at the psycho-energetic level, you are able to be in flow, as opposed to feeling like you are swimming against the current all the time. You stop being haunted by chronic fears, guilt, shame, anger, etc. You still experience those emotions at times but you are able to move through them with ease and grace, rather than have them as your default mode. You are also able to have a broader grasp of what is happening for others, which enables you to navigate your relationships with more understanding and compassion. You become more peaceful. Remember that you cannot have good health without inner peace (and you cannot have inner peace without addressing emotional toxicity). Internal harmony heals, which why people like Zen masters and Buddhist monks do not tend to get sick.

Before you proceed, I would like to invite you to set an intention for the experience you are about to have engaging with this book. For a moment, just ponder what brought you here, where you are right now, and where you want to be after you have done this work. Everything we ever change starts with an intention.

Please note that this books provides a multimedia experience and is accompanied by a variety of videos, audios and handouts. I will be referring to these additional resources as we progress through the book. You can find them at: https://dr-eva.com/shs-resources.

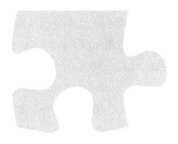

You Have More Control over Your Health Than You Realize

The Scientific Basis for the Health Sovereignty Solution Method

Many years ago, I learned first-hand how powerful your mind is in influencing your physiology. At that time, I was working while still studying, and my idea of managing stress was daily intensive exercise. No matter how exhausted I was feeling at the end of each day, I would gulp a caffeine drink or two and head to the gym, usually for a couple of hours of weight training followed by a high-intensity run or cycle.

This was long before I had a proper understanding of the fact that even though exercise is a healthy habit to have, it quickly starts working against you if you take it too far. I was absolutely taking it too far. At that point, I had a lot of unresolved trauma and was very easily emotionally triggered. It was not difficult for me to feel stressed to the point of feeling like I was not quite coping with life. I had very little resilience and so I was unknowingly abusing exercise as a way of trying to cope. Add to this long hours spent working and studying, and you have a perfect formula for your health to go pop.

So it did. I started experiencing some frightening symptoms, such as chest pains and being woken up with attacks of tachycardia (very fast heart rate) in the middle of the night. I also had my heart rate get stuck in higher zones following exercise. Increase in heart rate is absolutely normal while you are exercising, but after you have stopped, it should return to your resting levels relatively quickly. What started to happen was that 30 minutes after I finished running, my heart rate would still be double or more what my resting heart rate was at the time. This is an extremely bad sign because this can potentially lead to heart failure, stroke, or even sudden cardiac death.

At that point, I was in denial. Going to the doctor's meant admitting that something was wrong, and I refused to do that. However, I mentioned this to one of the lecturers at the Leeds Met university where I was studying at the time who specialized in exercise physiology and cardiac rehab. This was overheard by another physiologist, and they both started debating what could be wrong with my heart. After asking me some questions regarding my symptoms, they concluded that it was most likely supraventricular tachycardia. This is caused by abnormal circuitry in the heart that is usually present at birth.

As I was standing there listening to them, I felt like my world was ending. As they were saying this was probably a congenital issue, I was hit by this realization that my mother had a congenital heart problem! To make matters even worse, my mother's condition, despite her having symptoms for years, was not properly diagnosed until she was about 45 years old. Even though they were only theorizing and I had no medical confirmation of this, their assessment held authority with me, and it seemed like a fit because of the family history.

They demanded I go to see a doctor right away, so I did. I started my 24-hour ECG that day but I had to wait for other tests for a few weeks, including the one that would be able to tell me if there were any structural issues. I was absolutely terrified at the prospect of having this heart condition, which would essentially mean me having to be very careful and moderate my physical activity. *How am I going to cope with life if I could not do intense exercise?* I wondered. I literally concluded that my life was pretty much over if this problem were to be confirmed.

I was in a state of utter panic. My ECG was all over the place. The doctor asked me to do it multiple times and kept frowning at the results but refused to diagnose until seeing the results of the other tests. While waiting for those, I had multiple panic attacks per day. I would also wake up with panic attacks at night, covered in cold sweat. I was so fearful of what the tests would reveal that I could not function. Needless to say, being paralyzed with fear was making my heart symptoms worse, and the worse my symptoms were, the more panic I felt. A downward spiral that I know many people will relate to. After a week or so of having constant panic attacks and multiple episodes of tachycardia, I decided that I needed to do something. The appointments for those other tests were still weeks away!

I did some digging and made a decision to see a hypnotherapist. Even when going to see her, I had a panic attack when driving on the highway and had to pull over. My mind just would not stop creating all those doom and gloom scenarios and my body obliged adjusting my physiology to match my thoughts and emotions. I felt like I was going insane. The hypnotherapist was amazing, a very nurturing lady. This was my first ever experience with this modality, and after that first session, my panic attacks and my symptoms stopped. I never knew I was able to be that relaxed! She gave me the session recording and explained that I needed to change this automatic response I developed and how to do that.

Everything calmed down after that because I learned how to recondition that nervous system reaction, which, of course, positively impacted my physiology. I went to see her one more time, and that was all I needed to resolve this particular issue. I still had to heal all of my childhood and intergenerational traumas, but at that point, this was not on even on my radar. What was important to me at the time was that I had the tools and understanding to stop my panic attacks and my cardiac symptoms. The next 24-hour ECG came back normal. The results of the other tests came back absolutely fine too. In fact, the doctor who did my echocardiogram said I had a heart of a race horse. I never had that particular problem again.

Before I share with you the "how" of my method, it is critical that we are all on the same page with regards to how the mind-body-energy connection works. We have a number of sciences that show us very clearly and conclusively that we have an incredible amount of control over our health and our lives. Greater than most people realize or utilize. The application of these science that I will share with you throughout this book enables us to use this power. So let me first present you with a summary of why we want to apply the principles of quantum physics, neuroscience, epigenetics, and psychoneuroimmunology to our healing and everyday living.

All Healing Is Really Quantum Healing

Quantum physics is the main reason why somebody can have multiple traumas and be very emotionally toxic, or can have an autoimmune disease or cancer, and yet with the right motivation and application, this individual is able to not just restore their health but to thrive. Quantum physics teaches us that every material structure in the universe has a unique energetic signature. The surface you are resting on right now appears to be solid. As does the book you are holding in your hands. However, in reality, if you were to examine these seemingly solid objects under an atomic microscope, you would realize there is nothing solid there and that you are looking at empty space. This is because 99.999999999999 percent of an atom is made up of nothing. By "nothing" we mean no solid particles, but this "empty space" is actually made of a matrix of a wide range of frequencies that creates a field of information.

We perceive objects in our physical reality as solid because their particles are vibrating slowly enough to appear solid. This includes our bodies. The slower vibration (lower frequency and longer wavelength) means the particles appear in the physical reality for longer periods of time, but ultimately, it is all just energy and information. *Yes, that is very nice*, you might say, *but what on Earth does that have to do with health and healing?* And the answer is: EVERYTHING. Your thoughts, beliefs, perceptions, and emotions, which are energy, influence matter, i.e., your body and the rest of your physical reality. This means you will get the best healing results when you stop putting your faith in things and people outside of yourself and put it in the ability of your mind to influence your physical reality instead. This is true sovereignty.

So even though we are interested in root cause of illness and root causes of emotional toxicity, ultimately the mind-body-energy connection means that your mind can influence your body (matter) REGARDLESS of the origins of your health problem. The lower your vibration, the more you become solid matter. This makes you more vulnerable to the second law of thermodynamics (the law of entropy), that says that *left to itself, everything moves towards disorder and decay.* Disease is a low-vibrational state. On the flip side, the more you increase your vibrational frequency through positive emotional states, positive thoughts, empowering beliefs, etc., the more the cells of your body are more energy and less matter. This means your energy field is more coherent and orderly, which make you less susceptible to entropy and decay. In other words, disease states cannot be maintained. You can think of it as becoming immune to entropy. When I talk about energetic immunity, that is exactly what I mean.

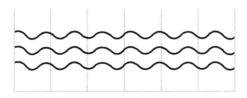

COHERENCE - HEALTH

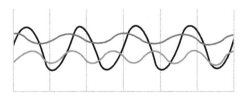

INCOHERENCE - DISEASE

COHERENT VS. INCOHERENT FIELD

Higher frequency and a more coherent energy field = health

Lower vibrational frequency and less coherent energy field = disease

Within the quantum field subatomic particles exist in infinite range of probabilities simultaneously. This right here is why in the anything is possible in the quantum field, why you create your own reality in every moment, and why if you choose to learn how to do it, you can affect your day-to-day reality to make sure it works for you!

Infinite number of probabilities existing in the quantum field mean we can manifest what we want into our physical reality. You choose. Something to be aware of though: if you create from the same level of mind (thoughts, beliefs, etc.) that created what you do not want (e.g., illness), you will continue to create the same undesirable reality. So, this may sound like a cliché, but in order to create a better reality for yourself, you have to increase the vibrational frequency of your thoughts, beliefs, emotions, attitudes, and perceptions. I am going to be sharing with you how to do this at every step of my method.

The quantum perspective points us towards the fact that the universe consists of independent energy fields that are entangled and interact with each other, meaning that interactions in the physical body are not just linear. Health becomes a lot more complex when you think about everything interacting together in a non-linear way. It is a very intricate matrix of communication. Critically, our psychological processes are absolutely involved in our health, as our thoughts, beliefs, perceptions, and emotions interact with the body in each and every moment.

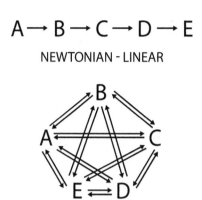

A → B → C → D → E

NEWTONIAN - LINEAR

QUANTUM - HOLISTIC

INFORMATION FLOW

The bottom line is that our cells actually communicate via the quantum field, so all healing is really quantum healing and goes far beyond chemical compound interactions in the body (such as hormones and neurotransmitters). Research by biophysicist Colin William Fraser McClare revealed that energetic signaling mechanisms, such as electromagnetic frequencies, are a hundred times more efficient in relaying information than hormones, growth factors, or neurotransmitters. To give you an idea of the difference, the speed of electromagnetic signals is 186,000 miles per second while the speed of a diffusible chemical is less than 1 cm per second. As astrophysicist Milo Wolff points out: *Nothing happens in nature without an energy exchange. Communication or acquisition of knowledge of any kind occurs only with an energetic transfer. There are no exceptions.* The newly emerging disciplines of quantum biology and biophysics embrace the study of quantum processes that underpin chemistry, but they are still considered "fringe" sciences from the mainstream perspective.

The most important take-away here is that the way our bodies work is very complex, and it goes far beyond biochemistry. Stress, trauma, toxic thoughts, people, and other toxic influences (e.g., mainstream media) all lower our frequency, which makes us more prone to disease. Again, our thoughts, beliefs, emotions, perceptions, and attitudes are energy, and they impact our epigenetic expression and cellular biology in a very powerful way. This energy is much more powerful than chemical messengers because the receptor sites on our body's cell surface are more sensitive to energy (frequencies) than they are to physical chemical signals. Ultimately, it is the unified quantum field that keeps us alive. The autonomic nervous system is the interface of this quantum intelligence, which is why balancing the autonomic nervous system is a key focus of this method.

So Why Is This Information Not at the Top of the Curriculum in Every School?

The simple answer is: money. The medical industry and Big Pharma, or as I call it, the medical mafia, have trillions of dollars at stake. Rockefeller medicine has nothing to do with healing. They treat symptoms. That is all. Their business model is about creating lifelong customers. If most people applied the principles I am discussing here to healing, then the multi-trillion-dollar drug industry would simply cease to exist. Do you not think that they are painfully aware of that? I assure you that they are. Hence, they go out of their way to program people to believe that the only way people can be free of disease is with the use of pharmaceuticals.

The fact is that the prevalence of medication use and polypharmacy in younger and older adults, as well as children, has increased dramatically in the last few decades. Every other commercial on TV in most Western countries is for some kind of pharmaceutical. If you look closely, most people in power are connected to Big Pharma in some way. Plus, those who are behind Big Pharma are the same people who train doctors (e.g., Rockefeller University) and dictate the world health policy via The World Health Organization. The same individuals are always at the top. If you care to research that, it will take you less than half an hour to confirm for yourself that this is the case.

At this point, I want to make clear that I am not against conventional medicine. There are times when we need medical interventions. When I broke my elbow in four places and needed an immediate surgery, I was very thankful for emergency medicine and all that it can do for us. Emergency medicine does indeed save lives. No arguments there. What I am against is brainwashing people to believe that they need drugs when they do not. Rockefeller medicine is completely inept at addressing chronic health problems. Just consider cancer treatments. With all the technology and advances available and trillions of dollars apparently going into cancer research, look at how useless these still are. Poisoning the body into health? That is their great idea? Is that really the best they can do?

And what about autoimmunity? Most people with autoimmune conditions are told there is nothing that can be done and they have to manage their illness with medications for the rest of their lives or cut the problematic parts of their bodies out! Really? Does that make sense to you? The patient is told that autoimmunity is their "stupid" body going wrong and attacking itself. This is completely ignorant, shows zero understanding of how the human system actually works, and it simply fails people. When I got my autoimmune diagnosis and was told there was nothing that could or needed to be done apart from being on medication, my answer was simple: *No, there might be nothing YOU can do. There is plenty that I can do to heal this.* So I did. Using these exact principles we are discussing here and throughout this book.

And what about people with chronic pain? Do you think they should just be prescribed painkillers with no effort made to get to the bottom of why they are in chronic pain in the first place? I do not. I consider that simply insane, particularly because those drugs are addictive and cause negative alterations in the brain. Do you see what I mean about creating lifelong customers? Drugs can offer a lifeline, but there should always be an effort to get to the true root cause, and in Rockefeller medicine there never is.

So why is conventional medicine useless at dealing with chronic health issues? Apart from the obvious already mentioned, which is money, their ongoing failures are due to their outdated conventional biology approach. This approach says that if there is a problem in the system, this can be attributed to one of the links along a linear reaction chain. So we give the body the replacement part (usually in a form of a drug of course) and expect all to be well, right? WRONG. As we know, all any drug will ever do is mask symptoms and give you some nasty surprises along the way in the form of side effects, which all drugs have. THERE IS NO TRUE HEALING involved in this process. I call the conventional medicine approach: *just cover things up and hope for the best.* That is why it fails people.

That is also what kills people, as demonstrated by the horrific number of iatrogenic deaths, also known as "death by medicine," every year, which goes into hundreds of thousands.

You would think somebody should realize by now that this is the true pandemic.

Dr. Bruce Lipton, a renowned cell biologist and one of the pioneers in the field of epigenetics, gives this analogy of having a fault light flashing on the dashboard of your car and going to the mechanic, who pretends to fix the car, but all he does is remove the bulb so that the flashing goes away. The customer thinks the car is fixed and drives off. How long before something in the car goes wrong? It is simply not a question of *if* but *when*.

Psychoneuroimmunology: How Your Mind Makes or Breaks Your Health

Decades of research have demonstrated that our mental and emotional states affect our immune and our endocrine systems, which, of course, has massive implications for healing. We can improve our immune function when we switch from stress activation, which many people experience chronically, to the relaxation response. This is why meditation, breathing practices, and other similar tools have been shown repeatedly by science to have a profound positive effect, not only on our mental but our physical health as well. Even looking at a flower creates a physiological response involving millions of nerve cells that can, in turn, create a positive or negative change in our physical body (depending how we feel about the flower)!

The science that aims to explain how our psychological health affects our immune function, and therefore our physical health and resistance to disease, is called psychoneuroimmunology. This phenomenon is a result of interactions via the sympathetic-adrenal-medullary axis (SAM axis), which involves the hypothalamic-pituitary-adrenal axis (HPA axis) and the sympathetic nervous system. Simply put, our psychological processes can either make us sick or make us thrive, depending on our response to what is going on internally and externally. Again, this is energy influencing matter.

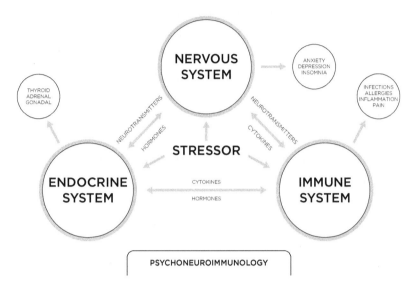

The field of psychoneuroimmunology research emerged after Ader and Cohen (1975) showed that immune system functioning can be conditioned. Since then, many fascinating studies have shown how various emotional states and social and behavioral factors influencing the brain can contribute to health, illness, and even death. Chronic anger, fear, anxiety, aggression, and hostility, as well as prolonged depression and untreated bereavement, are damaging to our health. They have been shown to negatively affect the activity and number of lymphocytes (white blood cells) that protect us from immunological threats. This means that chronic negative emotional activation can result in increased susceptibility to various infections, parasite infestations, as well as cancer cell proliferation. Notice that I am emphasizing the word "chronic." It is when those emotions are experienced in a chronic way that they become problematic. There is nothing wrong with experiencing them acutely, whereby if they show up, they are felt, we move through them, and they go away. Of course, chronic negative emotional states, chronic stress, and traumatic experiences can all be healed, which is the focus of this book. However, some people choose not to deal with those issues, and that definitely makes them more susceptible to poor health outcomes.

Right now, I want you to ask yourself what you have been taught about your body and health. What are you currently believing about your potential for healing? I ask because your answers will 100 percent determine your health outcomes. So, do you think that your body is defective? Do you believe that when you have symptoms that means something in your body has gone wrong? Do you believe that you need pharmaceutical interventions in order to maintain health? OR do you believe that the symptoms are only your body's way to communicate with you? That if you get out of the way, your body will heal because that is how it has been designed to survive?

Please understand that the body is not defective and stupid, as most people have been programed to believe. The body does not "go wrong" and it does not choose to attack itself out of nowhere, like in the case of autoimmunity! That is definitely not the case. There is nothing "wrong" with your body. Every minute of every day, your body is doing everything it can to heal and survive. It communicates what it needs with you. We need to listen. We need to give the body and mind what they need, and we need to get out of the way so the body can do the job it has been designed to do, which is to heal and thrive.

Going back to the mind affecting the body, at the end of the 19th century, an American psychologist William James said:

No mental modification ever occurs, which is not accompanied or followed by a bodily change. Later on Norman Cousins, the author of *Anatomy of an Illness* and *Head First: the Biology of Hope*, summarized this statement with three words: *Belief becomes biology.* What they both meant was that the body's physical reality can be altered by the more powerful reality of the mind; in other words, what is expected tends to be realized.

The Control Is in the Environment

Another empowering science with massive implications for healing is epigenetics. Until recently, we used to hear frequently that: *there is nothing you can do because it is genetic.* We know now that this is yet another outdated way of looking at disease and healing. Believe it or not, many doctors and patients are still playing the *blame the genetics* game. Those who like being victims love this narrative. That is OK. Some people are not ready to take responsibility, and we are not here to judge that. However, for anyone who wants to take control of their health, this science gives them that power because it clearly shows that we are not victims of our genes.

Epigenetics means the control is not in the genes but *above the genes*, which is what *epi* means. The bottom line is that if we optimize our mindset for healing and get all the dietary and lifestyle factors right, we have an incredible level of control over our health, which makes the relatively small genetic component much less significant. Studies on identical twins, such as the ones from Osaka University, demonstrate that it is not just genetics that dictate people's health outcomes. According to this research, identical twins, who, of course, share the same DNA, do not tend to manifest the same health issues.

There are, of course, diseases that are the result of one faulty gene, like Huntington's or cystic fibrosis. However, single-gene disorders affect less than 2 percent of the population, and even in these cases, optimizing the epigenetic factors, such as diet, lifestyle, and, of course, the mindset, will massively improve people's prognosis. In reality, the vast majority of people are born with genes that enable them to live a happy, healthy life. The diseases plaguing the world today, like heart disease, diabetes, autoimmunity, and cancer are NOT the result of a single gene but of complex interactions among multiple genes and environmental factors.

Dr. Bruce Lipton will tell you that scientists have linked many genes to many diseases but they have rarely found that one gene causes a particular disease. That is extremely rare. It is one thing for a gene to be linked to disease and another to cause disease. Dr. Lipton gives the example of a car key. Just because you need the key to start the car does not mean the car key controls the car or makes it drive. Another scientist summarized it this way: *When a gene product is needed, a signal from its environment, not an emergent property of the gene itself, activates expression of that gene.* In other words, the control is in the environment (diet, lifestyle, state of mind, etc.).

Geneticists working on the Human Genome Project had a bit of a shock when they discovered that the entire human genome consists of only 25,000 genes and not 120,000 as they had expected. This means there are simply not enough genes to account for the complexity of human life or human disease. There is a roundworm out there (Caenorhabditis) that has 1,200 cells and around 24,000 genes. The human body with fifty trillion cells contains only 1,500 more genes than that worm. Even though we have lipids and polysaccharides in our cells that serve very important cell functions, our cells are in the main an assembly of protein building blocks, and it is the changing of the proteins' electromagnetic charges that is responsible for their behavior, not DNA. Another reminder that we are electromagnetic beings!

So no, genes do not make us who we are and they do not ultimately control our health. DNA blueprints passed down through genes are not set in stone at birth. This is why the three pieces in the Triangle of Healing not only matter but make all the difference.

The Miracle of Neuroplasticity

Another field of study that I utilize in my method to a great extent is neuroscience. Apart from the understanding that neuroscience brings us with regards to why and how the techniques and exercise presented here work, we are utilizing neuroplasticity to remodel our neurology. Neuroplasticity is this amazing ability our brain possesses to adapt, change, and grow through reorganization as we learn new information. Neuroplasticity works by pruning (getting rid of neural connections) and sprouting (creating new neural connections). In a healthy brain these processes can take seconds.

As you are working through this book, you will have those "aha" moments, after which you will not be able to operate (think, feel, behave) in the same way as before. Those beautiful moments, when in an instant, the map of your world expands, are an example of neuroplasticity in action. What can also happen is that as new information comes into your awareness, suddenly what was appealing to you previously is not anymore. That can start the process of pruning some of the existing neural pathways.

Most of the time, however, the sort of transformations that most people are after when doing this work take time, awareness, and repetition. So just keep that in mind. Also, I want you to be aware that the initial moment of stepping out of your box is not always comfortable because we feel safer with familiarity, no matter how uncomfortable that is. If we persevere, we will be rewarded. That is why you need to be ready to change. If you are doing this because your mother or your partner thinks you should, you will likely step out of your box and pull right back. This is why it is so important that you are the one driving your process of change and you are positively motivated to achieve your goals.

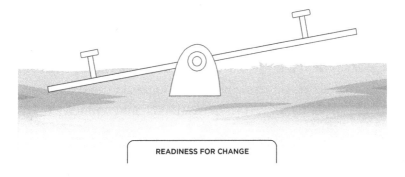

READINESS FOR CHANGE

Stem Cells – Embodiment of Pure Biological Potential

I would like to conclude this very brief review of sciences that show us how to take control over our health with mentioning the role of stem cells in healing. You can think of stem cells as the body's raw materials. All other cells with specialized functions are generated from stem cells. Under the right conditions, stem cells divide to form more cells called daughter cells. These then either become new stem cells (self-renewal) or become specialized cells (differentiation). Specialized cells have specific functions, such as blood cells, muscle cells, brain cells, immune cells, or bone cells. No other cell in the body has this incredible ability to generate new specialized cells, so stem cells truly are our allies when it comes to healing.

What is interesting, however, is that studies on wound healing show that being in stress-promoting emotional states (e.g., fear, anger) causes an interference in this process of stem cells becoming useful cells that can be utilized for specific purposes. This is because those emotional states activate fight-or-flight, or perhaps even freeze, response, which direct the body's resources to dealing with the threat, regardless of whether it is real or only perceived. In fact, this is the case every time we do not feel 100 percent safe and relaxed. In other words, at those times, the body is focused on surviving only, and any other processes, such as healing, are of secondary importance. Later in the book, we will talk more about optimizing your autonomic nervous system function for healing, but the above briefly explains why stress activation is not conducive to cellular regeneration and repair.

So, in summary, we can be in charge of our physical destiny if we choose to. There is enough scientific evidence to support this claim within these different scientific branches. I invite you to read on as we continue exploring how we can use the mind to dictate out health outcomes.

Why Your Subconscious Mind Rules Your Life

Many people confuse creating your own reality with positive thinking. Is positive thinking enough to create the physical reality and health that you desire? No. It is not. Why? Because in order to create positive physical reality using the power of your mind, your conscious (your thinking mind) and your subconscious (your emotional or feeling mind) have to be aligned. They have to be in agreement with each other. To fully understand this, you need to remember that it is your subconscious mind, not your conscious mind, that runs the show that is your life.

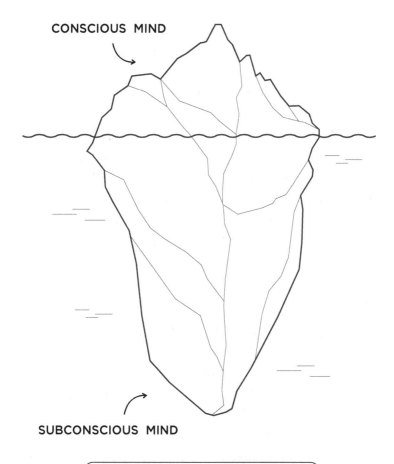

CONSCIOUS MIND

SUBCONSCIOUS MIND

REPRESENTATION OF THE
CONSCIOUS AND SUBCONSCIOUS MIND

The iceberg analogy has been used for many different concepts, but it just so happens that it explains the relationship between the conscious and subconscious mind perfectly as well. At the top, you have the visible part of the iceberg. No doubt it is powerful. If you have ever seen a huge iceberg like this in real life, you cannot deny it makes an impression. However, the majority of the iceberg is hidden underneath the water's surface. Just like the subconscious mind. The conscious mind is very powerful, no doubt about it. It is our thinking, logical, rational, creative mind. It is a home of declarative (explicit) memories based on knowledge and experience.

The subconscious mind is like the hard drive of your computer. It stores everything we ever experience. The subconscious mind is governed by feelings, rather than thoughts. It does not think; it reacts based on how it has been programed. It is a storage of stimulus-response records of whatever happens in our lives, as well as learned stimuli. It is habitual. This is the home of our beliefs and nondeclarative (implicit) memories based on conditioning, emotional reactions, and repeated experiences. Once something happens and we develop a behavioral response based on what happened, every single time a situation is repeated, or even remotely resembles that first experience, the subconscious will run that same pattern of behavior. That is how you develop fears and phobias, among other things.

The critical thing to remember is that when there is a battle between the conscious and the subconscious mind, the subconscious will win every single time.

An average person spends around 95 percent of their day running their subconscious programs and only 5 percent operating at their conscious level. Why is that a problem? Because the majority of most people's subconscious programs are a product of early exposure to stress, various traumas, and social engineering. Meaning they are predominantly limiting. Of course, not exclusively. Once you have learned to drive or play a musical instrument, these and many other activities become subconscious, which is very useful. However, most of your subconscious programs are limiting, which means you will struggle to create a positive reality for yourself.

When your conscious mind comes to the forefront, when you are more present, you can disengage this subconscious autopilot. In those moments, you have more control over your life, as that is when you are able to create the reality you truly desire. That is why you always hear how important it is to be in the now. Yet for most people it is extremely challenging to spend even a fraction of their regular day being truly present.

An average person has over 60,000 thoughts per day. The same thoughts lead to the same feelings and emotions, the same behaviors, and therefore, the same reality. This includes your biology. The same brain and body chemistry equals the same genetic expression.

So if you want something different, you need to step outside of that box. The cognitive aspect of choosing to change your thoughts is very important, but if you just do this, it will feel like hard work because of any limiting subconscious programs you may have. As I said, unfortunately, most people get hijacked by their limiting subconscious programs most of the time. So if you want your thoughts to be automatically more positive and more aligned with what you want, you need to address this holistically. You need to rewire your programming at the neurological level. This means healing your attachment adaptations, traumas, limiting beliefs, value conflicts, and so on.

When you look at every aspect of your reality: your health, your relationships, your finances, etc., and assess how happy you are with them, you will get an idea of much you need to rewire at the subconscious level in order to align your conscious and subconscious and create exactly what you want. That is not to say that you should not practice being present. You absolutely should. When you are able to connect to your body and create a sense of calm in the present moment, it helps you recondition your autonomic nervous system and accelerate healing. Besides, every moment is the only moment that exists and the only moment that is actually real. As humans, we spend most of our time in the past and the future, meaning we are constantly missing out on the now.

So How Do We End Up with These Negatively Conditioned Subconscious Programs?

Let me illustrate with an example. Imagine a child seeing a spider for the first time. The child is playing on the floor and has no concept of what a spider is. Then, the mother comes into the room, sees the spider, and in that moment, she freaks out, takes her slipper off, and starts screaming and bashing the spider. The child feels startled and fearful due to the mother's reaction. The child's subconscious says: *My authority that is Mom is scared and wants the spider dead. This means spiders are something to be scared of. They are dangerous. I AM NOT SAFE when a spider is around.* This program is now downloaded, and every time the child sees a spider, he or she will feel unsafe and fearful, maybe even to the point of having a panic attack or even passing out.

What if, instead, the mother came into the room and said: *Look, honey, this is a spider. Look at this beautiful creature. Isn't it clever? Isn't nature clever? Let's take the spider and put it outside.* Then, the mother gently takes the spider in her hand and removes it. In this scenario, the child marvels at the spider: *Mommy thinks the spider is wonderful, ergo I think the same.* The child is not going to be afraid of spiders and might even develop a special interest in nature and little critters. So this example shows you: 1) the function of the subconscious mind and how it becomes conditioned, and 2) the power of programming.

Now let us examine this further. So I said that in the battle of two minds the subconscious always wins. So consider this. This child is now a grown person with his or hers rational thinking fully developed, which they did not have as a small child. They see a spider and freak out; start screaming, sweating, their heart is racing. Their subconscious still tells them that they are not safe; spiders are to be feared. That is what got encoded in that original experience. However, as an adult, they say themselves: *Hang on a minute. I am a fully grown person and I am freaked out by a tiny spider.* They try to use their conscious mind to rationalize it, telling themselves the spider is not venomous, that they are bigger than the spider, blah, blah, blah... Yet next time they see a spider, they freak out again. The exact pattern of behavior repeats, regardless of how much they try to rationalize it and talk themselves out of it. It is automatic and it is instantaneous. Unless this issue is rewired at the subconscious level, this will keep happening.

If you ever had a phobia or fear of something, you will know exactly what I am talking about. The emotions take over, and the thoughts are not strong enough to counteract the feelings. This is precisely why talk therapy on its own (CBT, counseling, etc.) does not work when trying to address subconscious patterns. It is simply the wrong tool for the job. Do you know that children's toy where you have different shapes that you are supposed to push through the right shape holes? Using cognitive approaches to address subconscious issues is like trying to shove a triangular shape through a round hole and wondering why it is not working. If you could just talk your way out of having a subconscious problem, you would not be here reading this book and I would not have a thriving practice. We need to employ a range of techniques that will essentially help us rewire the brain, reprogram the mind, and rebalance our biofield in a coherent way. This is precisely what this method is all about.

So Why Is There This Difference in Reaction between the Conscious & Subconscious Mind?

The conscious and subconscious are two separate parts of the mind and they have different functions. Neurologically, the subconscious is your primal brain, which is focused on survival. So if something does not feel safe, your subconscious will try to "protect" you from it by producing certain emotional and behavioral responses, like in the example I gave earlier, even if this means making your day-to-day life miserable. The subconscious processes stimuli on the basis of whether a given response is conducive to survival or not. If a response had been previously employed and you survived, then that makes it valid to use again, regardless of how it may affect your current life.

Neurologically, the conscious mind is the newest part of the brain. This part of the brain is called neomammalian complex, estimated to have developed only a couple of millions years ago. Contrast this to the primal brain, estimated to have developed several hundred million years ago. In between those structures, we also have the paleomammalian complex (the limbic system) responsible for emotional processing. When there is an external stimulus to which our brain responds, that stimulus is read by our primal brain first. Speed is everything. Your primal brain is 900 milliseconds faster than your conscious brain, which is why very often you will react, and then it hits you a moment later that you have reacted.

For example, if I were to throw something at you, you would probably duck or catch it, and then a moment later, you would realize you had done that. Same when you drive a car and your primal brain detects a threat. You slam on the brakes without any conscious thinking, only to realize a couple of seconds later there was something in the road. If you had consciously thought about it, it would have taken too long, and you possibly would have ended up in trouble. So your primal brain reacts and then that impulse has to travel over fifty meters of neural pathways before it reaches your conscious awareness. So that it is why your subconscious, not your conscious mind, runs the show and dictates your behavior and responses.

The subconscious response is more of a reflex, like in the case with Pavlov's dogs. At first, the dogs heard the bell and their salivating was linked to the presence of food, but by the end of the experiment, they were so conditioned to salivate to the bell alone. This reflex cannot be helped until it is rewired. If we rewire our automatic survival-driven programs, we will start responding in the way that is conducive to living a happy, healthy life. We can then create this alignment between our subconscious mind and the conscious mind that is responsible for our wants and desires.

Once we have that alignment, we can create life and health we want to have. This congruence is critical. That congruent mind will then attract opportunities because you will be more tuned in to what you want and need and to what is going to serve you. You will then be able to take action without your mind sabotaging you and get the outcomes that you want. That congruence is what creates reality, not just positive thinking alone. The bottom line is that if you could get what you want with just positive thinking, you would not be reading this book. Creating your physicality is more complex than that, but if you have the right formula and put the work in, you can absolutely do it.

How the Belief Effect Determines Your Physical Reality

The power of the subconscious belief has been elegantly summarized by Henry Ford in this one statement that I am sure you have heard before: *Whether you think you can, or you think you can't—you're right.* The belief effect is another way to describe the placebo effect. We can also call it the perception effect or the expectation effect. As I am sure you know, placebo trials provide information whether a tested drug has any effect beyond that occurring when people take the actual drug. It is the patients' beliefs, perceptions, or expectations that a treatment activates their body's healing potential that creates the right biological response. Of course, in case of a placebo, that treatment is chemically inactive.

Our belief creates an expectation, and regardless of whether that is accurate or inaccurate, it equally impacts out physical reality. Note that the placebo effect, which essentially is your innate ability to heal, is probably the most researched phenomenon in science since all the control trials have a placebo group.

Yet this amazing phenomenon is quickly dismissed by people who say: *It is just a placebo effect.* Upon a brief mention of the placebo effect, medical students quickly progress to the "real" medical tools like drugs and surgery. However, if you bother to stop and think about what the placebo effect really means and how much power it means we have, it is truly something to celebrate.

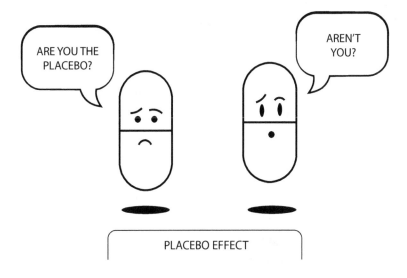

Everybody can utilize the belief effect for their healing, and I will be teaching you how to do this in this book. There are endless examples in scientific literature of how the mind affects the body and how the power of belief and intention can shape matter. Let us look at a few.

The Story of Mr. Wright

Back in 1957, psychologist Bruno Klopfer told the story of a man he referred to as "Mr. Wright," which was described in Klopfer's report entitled *Psychological Variables in Human Cancer.* You may have heard or read this story before because it is one of the better known documented cases of spontaneous remission, but it is one worth bringing back to your awareness before we start this journey together.

Mr. Wright had advanced lymphoma, and according to his doctors, he was dying. He had orange-size tumors in his neck, groin, chest, and abdomen. His doctors had exhausted all available conventional treatments and had given up on Mr. Wright. Around that time, Mr. Wright found out about a new experimental anticancer drug called Krebiozen. He begged his doctor to give him the drug, convinced that this drug would cure him. Mr. Wright was completely bedridden and fighting for each breath when he received the first dose of the treatment. He was given the injection on a Friday, and the doctors were convinced he would die before the end of that week. Much to everybody's surprise, by Monday, Mr. Wright was out of his bed, strolling around the unit, joking with the nurses. Klopfer reported that Mr. Wright's tumors had "melted like snowballs on a hot stove" because they had shrunk by half. Following ten more days of treatment, he was declared cancer-free and discharged from the hospital. The other patients who had received the same drug showed no improvement.

For the next two months, Mr. Wright enjoyed his cancer-free life. Unfortunately, he then became troubled by press reports questioning the efficacy of Krebiozen, which said the drug had no impact on lymph node cancer. This collapsed Mr. Wright's belief in the treatment. He became depressed, his tumors reappeared within a short period of time, and he was re-hospitalized. His doctors strongly suspected that Mr. Wright's initial positive result was due to the placebo effect. His doctor decided to lie and told Mr. Wright that despite the negative news reports,

Krebiozen was indeed effective and that the hospital had received a new improved batch of the drug.

Mr. Wright was very excited and agreed to proceed with the treatment. This time, the injection contained no drug whatsoever, but Mr. Wright believed he was being given the improved batch of the drug. Once again, tumor masses melted away, and Mr. Wright was shortly released out of the hospital. He remained cancer-free for another two months. Unfortunately, then came the report from the American Medical Association saying that Krebiozen was worthless and completely ineffective when treating cancer. Upon hearing the news, Mr. Wright relapsed once again, returned to the hospital and died two days later.

This is just one of many documented examples clearly showing that your expectations and beliefs can heal you or kill you.

A Genetic Skin Condition Healed with Hypnotherapy

In 1952, Dr. Albert Mason treated a genetic skin condition in an 11-year-old boy (ichthyosis). The doctor initially thought he was treating warts. He used hypnotherapy to treat the boy, and the skin became healthy. He had no idea he was treating a genetic condition. This transpired later. He believed the mind would tell the body what to do. The doctor believed it and the boy believed it, and that is exactly what happened.

Anita Moorjani Was Dying to Be Herself

Another case study of spontaneous cancer remission is that of Anita Moorjani, the author of the book *Dying to Be Me*. She had a four-year battle with cancer and went into a comma. Her family was told she was going to die. When in the coma, she had a realization that the root of her cancer was psycho-energetic.

When she came out of the coma, she started recovering very quickly and she now teaches about those mind-body relationships. She is free of cancer.

Glass of Cholera Anyone?

The germ theory states that microorganisms, such as bacteria, viruses, protozoa, or fungi, are the primary cause of disease. In reality, we now know that it is the terrain (the environment of the body), not the pathogen per sé, that determines what microorganism can survive in our body. If the germs were the main issue, we would all respond the same way, which is clearly not the case. Faced with the same pathogen, one person will get seriously sick or even die, whereas some other person will not even be aware that they had that germ in their system and that the body took swift steps to get rid of it. There are a number of factors that influence how susceptible somebody is to any pathogen and one of those factors is their state of mind and beliefs they hold.

In 1892, one of the critics of the germ theory, Bavarian chemist and hygienist Max Joseph von Pettenkofer, drank a glass of water containing a substantial amount of the bacterium that had been identified to cause cholera, *vibrio cholerae*. Amazingly, he was completely unaffected by the pathogen. When *Science* published an article about it, they said that for "unexplained reasons," the person was fine, but they still believed he was wrong to criticize the germ theory. Nobody bothered to investigate why he was unaffected by drinking a glass of something that was supposed to make him very ill or even kill him. The mainstream so-called science did not care.

Sham Procedures

Back in the 1950s, a sham surgery was used for patients with angina pectoris, which is characterized by recurrent pain due to decreased blood flow to the heart. Rather interestingly, the patients who received a sham surgery reported as much improvement in their symptoms as the patients who had the actual surgical procedure. Similarly, in the case of a sham therapy for back pain, an improvement of 40 percent was reported by the placebo group. In another sham surgery study from 2002, by Moseley and colleagues, the patients were divided into three groups. Two groups had different treatments for arthritic knees, and the third was the placebo group, which received a fake knee surgery. In this study, the placebo group improved just as much as the other two groups.

They Say Prozac, We Say Placebo

Most people are shocked when they discover that 80 percent of the effect of antidepressants has been attributed to the placebo effect. In addition, psychotherapy and placebo treatments show a lower relapse rate than that reported for antidepressant medication. Back in 1998, Dr. Irving Kirsch conducted a meta-analysis of 19 randomized, double-blind clinical studies evaluating the effects of different antidepressants. More than half of the clinical trials showed that the difference between the response to the drug and the placebo was clinically meaningless. Yes, it was that small. Some of those studies measured brain activity of the participants, showing real changes in the prefrontal cortex activity as a result of the placebo. Meaning those patients believed they were getting the actual drug. Dr. Kirsch then invoked the Freedom of Information Act to get access to unpublished clinical trials. He performed another meta-analysis, this time of 35 clinical trials on four widely used antidepressants. This analysis involved 5,000 participants and yet again it showed that the placebos performed the same as the drugs 81 percent of the time.

Saline for Pain

Placebo has been found to be more effective at treating pain than morphine in many studies over the last few decades. In fact, already during WWII, when there was a shortage of morphine, medics would use saline and operated on soldiers as if they had given them morphine. Soldiers who were convinced they were getting morphine felt little pain during those surgeries.

Some other conditions in which placebo treatments have been scientifically demonstrated to have a high rate of activity include: insomnia, hypertension, diabetes, ulcers, anxiety, high cholesterol, cough, asthma, sarcoma, dermatitis, headaches, rheumatoid arthritis, radiation sickness, inflammatory bowel disease, multiple sclerosis, Parkinson's, and cancer.

So How Does the Placebo Actually Work?

Dr. Joe Dispenza, the author of *You Are the Placebo* and *Breaking the Habit of Being Yourself*, talks about three key elements that come into play: conditioning, expectation, and meaning. By conditioning he means associating something with a physiological change as a result of experiencing that change many times before, e.g., taking a pill for a headache. If you then replace that pill with a placebo, the conditioned response will still cause the change in physiology and the pain will go away. Additionally, the placebo effect can occur if you have a reason to anticipate a different outcome because perhaps somebody you trust tells you that you can use something else to get rid of your headache. If you believe that enough, the body's physiology will be altered to fit in with your expectation. Finally, if you give something meaning because, for example, you have been educated about its benefits, you put more focus on it and make it happen. Because you have assigned this thing more meaning, you are more intentional about changing your inner state. You amplify your belief, so you amplify the belief effect.

I want to emphasize that the placebo effect is not just about the mind. It is energy (thoughts, beliefs, perceptions) influencing matter (the body), which leads to physiological changes. This includes changes in the levels of endorphins, neurotransmitters, such as dopamine and serotonin, as well as brain wave patterns. Norman Cousins said: *The process works not because of any magic in the tablet but because the human body is its own best apothecary and because the most successful prescriptions are filled by the body itself.*

The interesting thing is that even people's expectations about the effects of drinking can be more powerful in terms of predicting behavior than the actual impact of alcohol. In other words, drinking a placebo can produce all the physiological effects associated with drinking alcohol provided that the expectation is present. The same has been observed with drugs, such as LSD.

Another example is walking across hot coals. The stones' temperature should cause severe burns, yet thousands of people have done it without any negative consequences. Those whose belief collapses halfway through do get burned and need medical attention. There have also been studies done in which people imagined exercising or playing a musical instrument and through that mind training they were able to actually make physiological and neurological gains. I experienced this myself when I used to dance competitively. I developed a habit of practicing in my head and my dance coach would often comment how much I was able to improve in-between lessons. I was also able to maintain my skills quite well when being away on holiday because of mental rehearsals. Anybody who has ever tried to develop and maintain a skill or fitness knows how easy it is to lose your edge when you stop practicing or training for a few weeks. This was not that much of an issue for me, as long as I was disciplined enough to practice in my head multiple times per day.

In 2004, there was a study entitled: *From mental power to muscle power – gaining strength by using the mind.* In this study, participants imagined performing physical exercise and by doing that gained measurable improvements on the physiological level. The researchers concluded that the mental training employed in the study enhanced the cortical output signal, which drove the muscle to a higher activation level and increased strength.

Finally, what about all those people in their 90s who are very active physically and mentally sharp? The internet is full of videos of ninety-odd-year-olds dancing, doing yoga, and even running marathons. We are conditioned early on to believe that once you get to 50 – 60 years of age, it is all downhill from there. It is great to see that some people have escaped that ridiculous belief-engineering. Remember, they are not really special in any way. If it is possible for them, it is possible for you.

The Nocebo Effect

Naturally, we must also talk about the nocebo, as it is just as powerful. Nocebo is nothing else but the mirror-phenomenon to the placebo effect. This occurs when the expectation of a negative outcome produces the corresponding symptom or makes the symptom worse. This is, by the way, where many people who are sick shoot themselves in the foot. The human brain has this negative bias associated with survival and unfortunately, the same way we have the power to heal ourselves using the power of the mind, we also have the power to damage, or even kill, ourselves when we belief strongly that something is harming us. Below are some examples of how this works.

In 1982, a group of children in Japan who were allergic to poison ivy had one forearm rubbed with poison ivy, but they had been told the leaf was harmless. Then they had the other forearm rubbed with a harmless leaf, but were told it was poison ivy. All the children reacted to the harmless leaf with an actual allergic response, and 85 percent of children had no response on the arm actually rubbed by poison ivy.

Parkinson's patients who were told that their brain pacemakers (for deep brain stimulation) were to be turned off experienced dramatic negative symptoms even though the pacemakers were left switched on. There is also some consensus that Alzheimer's plague deposition is affected more by negative thinking than any other factors. This is because negative thinking alters the body's chemistry and results in upregulating gene expression that contributes to ill health and downregulates expression of genes associated with healing.

An interesting example of the potential nocebo effect is obtaining informed consent from patients before administering treatment. This disclosure of information about potential complications, or side effects of a treatment, if handled badly may trigger the nocebo effect. In other words, patients' awareness of the potential side effects may create an expectation, which, in turn, may produce the corresponding symptoms. In one study evaluating the effects of a new form of chemotherapy, 30 percent of people in the placebo group lost their hair, as they had an expectation that hair loss would occur. I used to know somebody who, when she had got diagnosed with breast cancer, absolutely refused to be told by her doctor about any side effects of the treatments they were going to use. She said she did not want to know because this was not going to apply to her, and she was going to be fine. She received chemotherapy and told me how every time she would go to have a treatment, she would meet other patients who all had horrendous side effects, such as nausea, hair loss, and so on. Her belief was that because she had never been told about the side effects, because she would not let her doctor talk about it, this was not part of her experience. Remarkably, she did not experience any side effects of chemotherapy.

Another issue that is frequently overlooked is the way in which patients are given diagnoses and how that impacts their ability to overcome illness. Many medical professionals still demonstrate a complete lack of awareness of just how much power they hold over their patients' well-being. Depending on how certain information is communicated, it can either empower the person and make them believe they can overcome their illness, or it can take away all their hope and consequently make them give in to the illness.

When a patient considers their doctor to be their ultimate authority, the statement: *you've got X months to live* is a terrible idea. It holds a lot of power. There are many cases of people dying almost exactly on their "expiry date" as announced by their doctor. It is my opinion that this is a very dangerous practice, and quite frankly criminal, particularly because doctors frequently get things wrong, as demonstrated by hundreds of thousands of iatrogenic deaths every year. The statistics speak for themselves. People surrendering their power to a white coat is a true human tragedy.

There was this famous case in 1974 of a man diagnosed with esophageal cancer. Every doctor around him believed the cancer was 100 percent fatal. They gave him a few weeks to live, so he died few weeks following his diagnosis. His post-mortem showed he did not actually had esophageal cancer. In fact, he did not had cancer at all! He had been misdiagnosed. His physician admitted that he did NOT die from cancer. He died because he BELIEVED he had terminal cancer. In my opinion, the word "terminal" should never be used when giving a diagnosis. It simply programs people to die.

Just pause and think about it for a moment. Our neurology is so powerful that a simple belief can produce a healing effect, but if that belief is negative, it can make us sick, or kill us. Irrespective of what others believe or present us with, it is vitally important that we take responsibility for influencing our own health in the way that we want to. Sending the right messages to our subconscious mind regarding how we feel about ourselves, our lives, our health, and our potential for healing our bodies is the first step to take. If we do not take control and program our minds, other people will do it for us. Only then, the chances are it will not be to our liking. So we have to make sure we program our minds for healing. The truth is that the most powerful resource we all have is our mind, so why not use it to our advantage? Persistent negative thoughts and emotions make us unhappy and sick, while a positive, nurturing mindset is the key to being happy, healthy, and full of energy. It is our choice which path we choose to follow. It may take some work, but it is definitely worth it!

Action Points:

1. Consider your situation. If you have ever been given a diagnosis, how were you informed? Think about the way the information was presented to you and how that affected your belief about the condition and your ability to overcome it. Did you feel empowered or victimized? Maybe you have never got a diagnosis but may have been researching your symptoms on the internet. The same applies. How did you feel when reading the information? Positive or defeated?

2. Based on those or any other experiences, answer the following questions and score your answers on a scale of 0 to 10 (0 being nothing at all/not at all, 10 being the maximum it can be):
   1) *Do you believe you are able to shape your physical health using the power of your mind?*
   2) *At this moment how strongly do you believe you will be able to achieve the health you want?*

   Write the answers down and when you get to the end of this book, I would like you to ask yourself these questions again.

3. Set an intention for this book. Take a moment to just ponder what brought you here, where you are right now, and where you want to be after you have done this work.

Creating Your Reality with Affirmations & Imagery

Remembrance & the Power of Intention

Many years ago, when I got diagnosed with ME (I also had fibromyalgia), I was told by the doctors not to get my hopes up because only about 2 percent of people recovered fully from ME. I honestly do not know how accurate those stats actually were at the time, but I remember saying to one of the doctors: *That is fine. Two percent is good enough. I will be in those two percent.* I know many people hearing something like that would collapse under the weight of it, but I did not really feel like I had a choice. To me full recovery was the only option. Falling ill had pulled the rug from under my feet. Everything stopped. I was no longer living. I was barely existing, which is why I decided that I was either going to get my life back or I did not want to live at all.

At my worst, I was only able to be up for about a couple of hours per day, after which I was so exhausted I had to go back to bed. All I could do most of the time was rest and sleep, but, of course, because I had this all-over-body aching and discomfort, spending all these hours in bed was pretty torturous. Basically, I lost the ability to live an even remotely normal life, which I know many people who have had any of these conditions will relate to.

Prior to getting ill, I had really enjoyed running, weight training, and I danced competitively. Obviously, I was not able to do any of that anymore, as I struggled to walk slowly for more than five minutes on a treadmill. Still, I felt depressed and I had to do something proactive. So I decided to start with my five minutes and build it back up again. As a side note, that is where many people with chronic-fatigue-related conditions go wrong. They cut out the movement because it is so challenging to do any exercise. That is a huge mistake. Moving is an essential part of recovery from chronic fatigue and fibromyalgia.

Even though I could not do much physically, I spent time every day imagining myself running and dancing. I was daydreaming a lot, which as you may is a form of meditation. I actually would do my running visualizations to my favorite running music, and I would also practice my dance steps in my mind. The more I did that, the more positive I felt, and the more I believed that would run like I used to again. I worked on creating my new reality every day. I was also doing trauma work at that time and was using other strategies to get my health back on track.

In less than a year, I was running again. I also got back to doing dance competitions. What was interesting was that I did not really lose my dance skills, which you would expect under the circumstances. The mental rehearsals kept the neural pathways nicely conditioned so when it was time to get back into it, within a few weeks of training, I was back where I had been before I got ill! This was quite a long time ago, and at the time, I did not understand the neuroscientific basis for what I had experienced. These days we have a better insight into why and how this works. You should never underestimate what you can achieve, provided that you are prepared to actively engage with the process of creating and maintain the required consistency to get to where you want to be.

Time to Remember Who You Really Are

All possibilities exist in the quantum field, and you can choose what version of reality you want to merge with. Your subconscious mind does not know the difference between your current reality and any of your future timelines. As we previously said, mind and matter are NOT separate. You create your reality in each and every moment, and the more present you are, the more choice you have with regards what you actually create for yourself. It is amazing to me how many people out there are still not on board with this concept! Imagine how the world would change in an instant if everybody was creating beautiful lives for themselves driven by their hearts.

Humanity has forgotten what their true abilities are, mainly due to sophisticated programming and mind control methods used in education and by the media. But since you are here, reading these words, perhaps you remember who you really are. A creator being. This is the true intelligence. Humans have been brainwashed that in order to be considered intelligent, you have to have a high IQ. I personally know quite a few highly "educated" people with very high IQs who are emotionally and spiritually handicapped, are very fear-based, and always attract what they fear into their lives. Well, guess what? They are also creator beings, but they create from the place of fear and zero awareness of how the mind works! In this current era of evolution in consciousness, they are going nowhere fast unless they choose to open their minds and hearts to the fact that we do live in a quantum universe.

The key reasons why people struggle to manifest what they desire are unresolved traumas and messed up belief systems. This is because that creates a neurological and emotional landscape that has an underlying vibration of fear, and when your subconscious is full of fear, it will always derail you to ensure you "stay out of trouble" and away from anything that could be "threatening" to your survival in any way. As we said, the subconscious does not know what is real and what is just in your mind so it will often overreact, just in case.

The Power of Intention

Before we progress to some more advanced practical techniques to help you manifest the health and reality that you want, let me just briefly talk about intention. In short, to initiate a positive change in your life, it is critical to set the right intention. From the work of many great people, such as Masaru Emoto or Lynne McTaggart, we know that our minds can affect not only our physical realities but also our external realities. Masaru Emoto's experiments, which you may have heard of, included the difference in the crystalline structure of water before and after prayer. One of his famous experiments was the Lake Biwa experiment.

In 1999, Dr. Emoto held a gathering of around 350 Japanese citizens, who had all offered their prayers for Lake Biwa, the largest freshwater lake in Japan. At the time of the gathering, Lake Biwa was a polluted and putrid-smelling mass of water. About a month after the prayers were offered, complaints about the lake had drastically decreased. The water condition improved significantly, and the foul odor disappeared. Dr. Emoto's water experiments can be found on YouTube, where you can see the changes in the crystalline water structure for yourself. I also recommend watching Lynne's Intention Experiment lecture from The Conference for Consciousness & Human Evolution (TCCHE).

So why am I bringing your awareness to setting the right intention before you even start this work? Because an intention is a guiding principle for how you want to be, live, and show up in the world. Having a clear intention will help guide your actions as you move through each day. An intention should not be confused with a goal. It is not something specific and tangible that you frame in time or evaluate. Goals are head-driven, whereas intentions are heart-driven. You want to absolutely have goals, but goals are not your starting point. An intention is. Your intention simply defines what you want to align with in your life. You can think of it more as an aim, a purpose, or attitude that you want to commit to.

Intentions evoke feelings and purpose, for example:
I want to open my heart and be more compassionate.
I want to be more courageous and express myself freely.
I want to feel more connected to people around me.
I want to feel more passionate about life.
I want to enjoy more energy and vibrant health.
I want to find balance and inner peace.
I want to unconditionally love and accept myself.

Setting an intention is a way to bring your heart and mind into alignment. When you put an intention out there, you set in motion the change you want to see in your reality. Naturally, your intention should be closely tied to your personal thoughts, values, and perspective on life. It should be positively focused. So, ask yourself, what would you like to build, create, or nurture in your life? What would you like to manifest in your reality? Before you continue, define your intention in order to set the manifestation process in motion while you are working through this method to transform your health. I do also recommend you set yourself some goals before you start. I have included a video on what to look out for when setting goals in the Additional Resources.

Accept Where You Are Right Now

When creating your new reality, you must acknowledge and accept where you are right now. This is very important. When you refuse to acknowledge where you are and you are in denial, you cannot move forward. You will be recycling the same old reality. The way your nervous system is conditioned will be reinforced, and you will continue to produce the same biology to go with that old conditioning. Because you are reading this book, you have clearly acknowledged, at least on some level, that your current reality is not satisfactory and you want to change it. So that, alongside setting your intention, is a great step forward.

Fully accepting where you are is just as important. You need to choose to be acceptant of where you are currently because otherwise, you create resistance. This is a problem because if you are resisting your current reality, you create more attachment to that which you do NOT want. You unknowingly make the reality you do not want stick around—what you resist will persist. When you resist and attach to where you are right now, to put it plainly: you put a noose around your own neck.

However, you do have a choice. You can choose to accept. You can choose to surrender to this moment. Surrender and let it be what it is in this moment. No attachment. It is what it is. Know that you have already started moving towards your new reality. Give yourself permission to choose to surrender with this knowing now.

The Dos & Don'ts
of Effective Affirmational Work

One of the most powerful ways to rewire the brain and create your own reality is using affirmations and mantras. Affirmations are simply statements that motivate, inspire, and encourage you to take action and realize your goals. When affirmations become embedded in your subconscious, and become your beliefs, they help you create a positive reality without you having to consciously focus on it all the time. Mantras tend to be much shorter than affirmations, often a word or two of special significance. Mantras can also be sounds, but for the purpose of what we are doing here, we will focus on words.

It is worth noting that using affirmations effectively is a bit of an art, so I want to share my top tips with you to help you create yours in the most powerful way. In addition, I will introduce you to a very powerful modality that forms the backbone of my method and will help you significantly accelerate the consolidation process. This means that rather than spending four to six weeks installing affirmations into your neurology, you can achieve it in one to two weeks. The exact time does depend on your existing beliefs, frequency with which you do affirmational work, and whether a given affirmation is connected to your identity. But, on average, I find it takes a quarter to a third of the time you would otherwise have to commit to achieve the same result. You will notice this about me as you continue— I do like efficiency!

The modality is called Havening Techniques®, also known as Delta Wave Techniques or Amygdala Depotentiation Techniques. It is a psychosensory treatment that uses simple touch to permanently eliminate unwanted feelings from distressing memories and events. In addition, this modality is extremely useful for promoting self-growth, as it can be used to plant positive concepts within the brain. The method, created by Drs. Ronald Ruden and Steven Ruden, is derived from and consistent with current neuroscience literature. Havening Techniques® is easy to learn, can be self-applied, is rapid, gentle, and has no side effects. I am including an eGuide that tells you more about how Havening Techniques® works, its applications, and how to use it in the Additional Resources.

So let us first look at those important rules when working with affirmations.

Phrase Your Affirmations Positively

This is because the subconscious mind understands and is able to process direct experiences but not language. For example, the subconscious does not understand negation, which is a function of language. There is no direct experience of the word *not*, so the subconscious cannot make sense of it. Only your conscious mind can. So if your affirmation is *I am not stressed*, your subconscious will focus on what it can make sense of, something that you have had previous experience of. In case of the statement *I am not stressed*, it is going to be the word *stressed*.

This means that if you keep repeating *I am not stressed* over and over, you will make yourself more stressed. Your subconscious will then create the biology to go with it. In this case, we can reframe this statement to *I am relaxed, I am peaceful*, or whatever the opposite of *stressed* is for you.

Use Present Tense

The subconscious has no concept of past or future. In the quantum field, time as we understand it on the conscious level does not exist. Everything just is. Past, present, and future are happening simultaneously. The subconscious operates in this way. Only your conscious mind understands time. So the best way to communicate with your subconscious is to state things as though they are happening right now. This also engages the conscious mind and helps us to more quickly accept that affirmation as our "new truth" on both the conscious and subconscious level. There is no point in saying, *I will be relaxed at some point in the future*. This is far too vague. It is much more effective to say, *I am relaxed*, or *I am healing right now*. I also recommend expressing gratitude for what you are wishing for as though it is a done deal, so to speak, for example, *I am grateful for my body healing in each and every moment*.

Bring in a Visual Aspect

If your affirmation is *I am becoming healthier every day*, you need to think about what that looks like for you. This helps your subconscious build a more accurate picture of what you actually want to achieve. So, for example, there are certain things you might be able to do when you become healthier that you were not able to do before, such as exercising. So you create a visual that goes with each of your affirmations. This is particularly important when your affirmations are ambiguous, in other words, when you use words in your affirmations that may have more than one meaning. You may use the same visual for multiple affirmations.

Use Emotive Words as Much as Possible

Your subconscious connects best with words describing feelings and emotions. This is the language of the subconscious, so make sure that your affirmations evoke positive emotions in you: *I am free, I am powerful*, etc. I highly recommend that you avoid words, such as *pain, stress*, etc. Even if you say: *I want to be free of pain*, the most emotionally charged word here is still *pain*, and your brain will connect with that first. So you want to think of the opposite of being *free of pain*, for example being *comfortable*. On the energetic level, high emotional charge means that you emit a higher vibrational frequency and you attract more of those similar vibrations.

If You Need to, Use Gradation

This is very important and the reason why many people dislike affirmational work. People often tell me that saying certain affirmations makes them feel like frauds, or that it makes them cringe. Let me explain. For somebody with poor self-worth who lacks self-love, jumping straight into *I love myself unconditionally* is too big a jump. They are not quite ready for that, which means their subconscious will throw resistance at it. It is like trying to jump from one bank of a really wide river to the other. This is why I have had many people over the years telling me they did not get on well with EFT, and this is because many practitioners do not understand that they need to grade the affirmations depending on where their clients are.

70

So when *I deeply and completely love and accept myself,* or any other affirmation, is a step too far, I recommend grading your affirmations. It is the equivalent of having some stepping stones so you can get to the other side of the river more easily. What does that look like? If you are currently not able to look yourself in the eye in the mirror and say: *I love you just the way you are,* then start with something less intense, for example, *I recognize I have positive qualities.* If you can look in the mirror, say those words, and not feel like you want to throw up, you are good to go.

Next, you stay with that affirmation for a week or so until it feels completely natural and true. Then you change it to, for example: *I am now starting to approve of myself,* or whatever is acceptable to you. Again, continue affirming that until it feels completely natural and becomes your new truth. Then you can progress to saying to yourself: *I like and accept myself because I am a good person* or something like that. Eventually, you will be able to say: *I love and accept myself unconditionally* without that subconscious resistance that you would have had if you had started with that. So if you need to, you can use less intense words to start with, or you can use phrases such as *I am now starting to...,* etc. As long as you feel neutral and do not get a strong negative visceral response, you are in the right place. From there, it will not take you long to progress to those more intense statements.

Affirmations You Use Must Resonate with You

For affirmations to work, they MUST resonate with you. This is why even though I will be giving you affirmations you can work with, I always encourage clients to create their own. I will give you many examples throughout, as we use affirmations

71

to achieve different therapeutic outcomes, and you can use them as they are, provided they resonate with you. If not, use your own words to create ones that do resonate.

Repetition Is Key

This is extremely important. You did not develop the beliefs you have because you heard something once, or something happened once. Whether it is a belief, such as: *It is bad to be late* or *I am not good enough*, its consolidation required repetition. So now to rewire your brain to create the reality you want, you need to use repetition as well. Just repeating an affirmation once or twice is not going to do anything. This is why I recommend you start with this work right away so that by the time you have finished working through this book, you will have, at least in part, changed your subconscious programming and your reality will hopefully start to look different as a result.

So again, it is all in the repetition. I cannot emphasize this enough. Why do you think you see the same commercials over and over? Why do you think politicians use the same phrases over and over? These are very powerful ways to program your mind. If you do not take control of this process, I absolutely guarantee that you will be programed by other people, and you will live your life according to what they have programed you with. If you want to be in control, you need to put some work in, but it is worth every moment you spend on this.

Different Ways of Using Affirmations

Affirmational Havening®

This is by far one of the most effective and fastest ways to consolidate your affirmations neurologically. When using this method, you apply gentle stroking to your face, arms, and palms (see diagram). This touch produces an electrical brain wave called a delta wave, which is the same brain oscillation that dominates in deep sleep, or when you feel extremely relaxed. The associated neurochemistry is very healing to the mind and the body. One of those neurochemicals that Havening® boosts is oxytocin, known as the love and social connection hormone. Many organs in the body, such as the intestines, the heart, and the liver, as well as the immune system have been found to contain oxytocin receptors. This makes those organs more receptive to oxytocin and its healing effects.

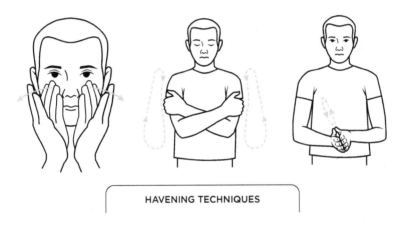

HAVENING TECHNIQUES

When you apply Havening Touch®, there is no sequence. You can stroke your arms, hands, and face in whatever order you want to, however many times you want, and change between them as you choose to. I would like to invite you to follow along with my Affirmational Havening® video in the Additional Resources to make sure you can learn this technique properly and use it with confidence. In this video, I give you examples of affirmations you can use to calm down your nervous system.

Even if you do not fully connect with all of these statements, just give yourself permission to go along with it the first time. You can then adjust the statements to suit you, as we discussed before.

Once you are comfortable using Affirmational Havening®, I would like you to pick a handful of affirmations that are most important for you right now and spend 5 to 10 minutes every day havening in front of the mirror. That way you are going to get an additional effect due to the mirror neuron activity. Mirror neurons are a type of sensory-motor cell located in the brain that is activated when you perform an action or you observe another person performing the same action. So the neurons "mirror" the action of the other person, as though the observer were performing that action. In this case, that other person is you, as you are looking at yourself in the mirror. This means that you get double the effect from the action you are performing, which helps the positive programing take effect even faster. This is what I call efficiency.

Writing Your Affirmations Down

Some people write affirmations or mantras on post-it notes and stick them around the house. This is fine because every little bit helps, but my recommendation is that this is done in addition to Affirmational Havening®. If you use post-it notes, remember that your brain does get used to things quickly, and then you gloss over them. If you want it to be more effective, use bright colors, put the notes in places where you have to look at them, and remember to change them and move them around frequently.

It is also a good idea to write your affirmations daily in your journal. When we write affirmations down, we activate our Reticular Activating System (RAS). The RAS is an attention

74

filter and basically explains why we get what we focus on. It finds ways to trigger your alertness to the things that you center your attention on, or as the Greek philosopher Epictetus said: *You become what you give your attention to.* So if you focus positively, soon you see positives in everything. Because your RAS keeps you centered on your outcomes, it encourages you to take positive steps towards achieving them. You can think of the RAS as the gatekeeper of information that is admitted into the conscious mind, connecting the conscious and the subconscious. Normally, incoming information is processed and analyzed in the hippocampus, which is a section of the brain responsible predominantly for the consolidation of information from short-term to long-term memory. Then the brain decides what to store in the long-term memory. This is why when designing affirmations and visualizations that we want to become our reality, we want to be creative with our imagery to ensure the right images are imprinted or encoded. Writing things down and saying things out loud helps that encoding process, as does Havening® because it acts on the hippocampus.

Using Mantras

Another thing you can do is to repeat your key mantras over and over as you are doing something else, e.g., washing dishes, cleaning, etc. Because your hands are busy, you cannot use Havening Techniques®, but you can treat washing dishes, or some other chore, as part of your mindfulness practice and add mantras as part of that process. In this case, I recommend picking three to five short statements that you repeat over and over, for example, *I am calm, I am strong, I am resourceful, I am resilient, I always find the way.* So you repeat those over and over. Obviously, if these do not work for you, create your own. Some people use mantra beads, which is great, but for the reasons we already discussed, if your hands are available, you may as well use Havening® to maximize the results. If you want to use mantra beads, ensure that you actually put yourself in a state of meditation because those lower brain oscillations (delta, theta, alpha) are essential for planting those new concepts and consolidating them neurologically.

Powerful Imagery Tools to Help You Achieve Your Outcomes

Imagery is another tool that I encourage you to start using right away to create the reality you desire. Before we proceed, let me clear up a few things. Firstly, everybody can visualize; otherwise, you would not be able to recognize your own house, and you would be buying bananas when you really want to buy apples. In fact, dreams are nothing more than visualizations. There is this very rare condition called aphantasia, which refers to the inability to conjure mental images. Researchers from the University of Chicago conducted a study on this during which they showed photographs of three rooms to dozens of individuals with both typical and limited imagery. The participants were asked to draw the rooms, once with the help of a picture and once from memory. Even though they found that people with aphantasia could place only a few objects in the room and their drawings were simpler and less detailed, compared to the other group, they still managed to perform this task! The researchers concluded that people with aphantasia lack visual imagery, but they appear to have spatial memory. This is different from visual imagery and may be stored differently, but who cares? The bottom line is that even people with this very rare condition can use imagery to create their reality. When doing imagery work, we do recruit all the senses anyway.

For purposes of clarity, it is true that visualizing comes easier to some people than others. If you are a person who learns best with visual input, you will find visualizing very easy. If you are naturally more of an auditory or kinesthetic learner, you might find creating pictures in your mind more challenging, but as you do it more, you get better at it, and vice versa. Highly visual people may be more challenged when it comes to kinesthetic activities. I am a highly visual person, what you would call a "nuclear visual," yet I was able to master ballroom and Latin dancing to a very high level and win multiple national competitions. It did not exactly come naturally to me at first. I remember being quite confused during my first ever Waltz class! Remember neuroplasticity? That is why you are able to get really good at something that may not come naturally to you at first.

Imagery Practice

Before I take you through a practical exercise, I want to emphasize that unlike your conscious mind, your subconscious mind does not differentiate between reality and fiction. That is the reason you can use imagery to create real physiological changes in your body. The first step in intentional self-healing is to realize and experience first-hand that your mind affects your body. Read the paragraph below slowly to give yourself an opportunity to create relevant imagery that engages all the senses. As you are reading, be mindful of any bodily sensations and emotions that you might be experiencing.

Imagine that you are walking along the street in a small, picturesque town. It is a nice sunny day. The temperature is very pleasant. It is just right. On your right-hand side you have a river. On your left there is a row of shops. You spot a cake shop with a very elaborate window display, so you cross the street and head towards it. You stop by the window for a moment to marvel at the beautiful display. As the cakes are baked on the premises, you can smell the most amazing aromas coming from the inside. You have not eaten for most of the day, as you have been busy sight-seeing, so you decide to step into the shop and get a slice of one of their amazing cakes. As you wait in line, you are immersed in the enticing aromas. Deciding what to have is challenging because the whole display looks delicious. Finally, it is your turn, and you make a selection. You cannot wait to take a bite of your chosen cake. You leave the shop, cross the street and sit on a bench by the river. You unwrap your cake and take a bite. At first, you taste the intensity of the flavors and you praise yourself for choosing well. Then, you sense something slightly chewy. You swallow and take another bite. Again, it tastes chewy and slightly off. You decide something does not feel right, so you spit the cake into a serviette, only to realize that inside the cake was a big juicy worm and that you had just eaten half of it.

Before you say this was mean of me, I would like to remind you that there is no cake and there is no worm. All of this was in your imagination. If you nonetheless experienced any bodily sensations or emotions, this tells you that you are more than capable of using your mind to influence your body. Perhaps you felt the sun on your face? Perhaps the imagined aromas of the cakes made you produce some saliva or made you feel hungry? Perhaps the imagery reminded you of something from the past, or somewhere you had been before, and you felt an emotion? Maybe you were looking forward to your cake and felt surprised, disappointed, or even disgusted that there was a worm in it? The bottom line is that your mind produced some imagery that then produced associated feelings and perhaps emotions, which actually had an impact on your biology.

If you had no effect at all, this means that you either tend to cling to control, you have a level of disconnect between your mind and your body, or you simply did not connect with the words on the page but may have had a different result if you were able to listen to the description. Whatever it is, it is fine. We will be addressing the first two issues with this method. I do actually have another exercise (Lemon Imagery) that I invite you to do. You can find it in the Additional Resources.

Future Outcome Havening®

We have already discussed Havening® as a method, and I hope that you have watched my Affirmational Havening® video. If not, I really encourage you to do that and to start using Affirmational Havening® daily or as frequently as you can. Future Outcome Havening® is another variation of this modality that goes very well with what we have been focusing on in this chapter. I do have a dedicated video in the Additional Resources that takes you through Future Outcome Havening®.

The premise is very simple. First, think about something you want to achieve. This has got to be important to you and must create a positive emotional response. Otherwise, it is unlikely to work. Once you have decided, create a movie in your mind of what it is you want to achieve as if you have already achieved it. Start applying Havening Touch® (i.e., stroking your hands, face, or arms). Continue to haven as you are creating your imagery, adding as much detail to this scene as you can. Make it dynamic, vivid, and colorful. I talk through this process

79

in more detail in the video, so again, please watch! Do this for 5 to 10 minutes every day.

Please know that this takes practice. Your mind will keep going on tangents, and you may find yourself thinking, analyzing, arguing with yourself inside your head, stressing, obsessing, and "efforting." If this happens, just bring your mind back to your outcome, over and over. Patiently. Without getting annoyed. Without judging yourself. It gets easier and easier as you do it more. Most people will start with only being able to stay present for a few seconds before their mind starts to distract them. Please be OK with that. Do not get attached to any expectations. Continue to practice to build it up. Some days this is going to be easier than others.

Finally, remember there is a difference between wanting to achieve an outcome and being too attached to the outcome, or being obsessed with an outcome. When you are too attached, again, you create resistance. You end up trying to force it and you are actually in a fight against whatever it is that you are wanting to change. So it is about being emotionally activated by the outcome but having trust that this is already happening in another NOW moment (all possibilities occurring simultaneously). So there is no need to try too hard. It is about letting it happen, letting that desired reality merge with your current one, without being too controlling and obsessive about it.

Vibrant Health Havening®

There is another variation of creating your physical reality with Havening® that I want to share with you. I have called it Vibrant Health Havening®. This involves spending a few minutes per day, again applying Havening Touch®, recalling the time in your life when you were at your best with your health. If you are one of those people who has always had health challenges, and maybe you have never had optimal health, simply pick a time when you recall being healthier, more energetic, and more resilient than you are now. Any improvement on where you are currently is still a positive step in the right direction.

Much like in Future Outcome Havening®, you want to be applying Havening Touch® throughout while creating a vivid, colorful movie of that time. Recall as much detail as you can. What is happening? Where are you? Is there anyone there with you? Remember to be in your own body; in other words, connect with what is happening in that memory through your own eyes. Notice what you are seeing, hearing, and feeling. What are you saying to yourself? If there are other people involved, what are they saying? Connecting with positive emotions is critical with all of these techniques I am teaching you. The body does not know the difference between an emotional response created by an actual experience and an emotional response created by a thought. However an emotion is produced, it will alter the body's physiology and biochemistry. This works both ways, of course, whether it is positive or negative. It is the same with fear, anger, anxiety, etc. The body will respond with stress chemistry whether a threat is real or perceived.

When I was very ill and played movies in my mind of myself running again, this is exactly the technique I was using, except back then, I did not know about Havening Techniques®. There was a study back in the 80s in which elderly men were asked to spend five days recalling their past. One group was asked to just reminisce about the earlier years, and the other was asked to actually pretend they were 22 years younger than they actually were. The environment they were in for the duration of this experiment was set up to make that easier for them. The physiological tests taken at the end of the experiment showed their bodies were structurally and physiologically younger. The changes were slightly more pronounced in the group that pretended to be younger, but certainly the first group did show significant physiological improvements. Like I said, when creating this imagery, you have the additional impact of Havening®. However, if you wanted to further amplify your results, think of any behaviors from that time of your life when your health was better that you could imitate now.

Action Points:

1. Practice Affirmational Havening® for 5 to 10 minutes per day in front of a mirror. You can either use the affirmations I have offered or design your own. To begin, pick a handful to work with. You can write them on a bit of paper and stick it to the mirror to help you remember what you are working with.

2. Spend 5 to 10 minutes per day practicing Future Outcome Havening® or Vibrant Health Havening®. You can alternate between them or pick the one you prefer.

3. Listen to the Vibrant Health meditation available in the Additional Resources (https://www.dr-eva.com/shs-resources), ideally every day for 4 to 6 weeks.

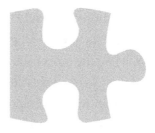

Self-Awareness as the Main Key to Your Success

Emotional Toxicity & Secondary Gain

I used to know somebody who, to an untrained eye, may have appeared to be the unluckiest person in the world, but in reality, what she was experiencing had nothing to do with luck. We already discussed in Chapter 1 how we create our own reality in each and every moment. I advocate taking responsibility for what we create, but this only works if a person is self-aware enough to recognize they operate in victim mode and, of course, if they are willing to take action to change that. Unfortunately, this lady had one of the most extreme cases of what I call chronic victimitis that I have ever come across, and yet she was completely unaware of it.

She kept saying that her children were her whole life. The problem was that her children were entering adulthood at the time and had less and less time for her. The more they tried to live their own lives, the more she would attract all sorts of unfortunate events to herself, which would then made them stay close and fuss over her. She had the most bizarre "accidents," always at the exact time that her children were scheduled to be away from home. In a matter of months, she chopped her fingertip with a knife, she had three car accidents, each of them associated with minor injuries that required hospital visits, somebody pushed a trolley into her in a supermarket and damaged a tendon in her foot, and she fell down the stairs. None of those resulted in any serious damage. It was just enough to get attention from her children. I was, however, concerned that she may end up in more serious trouble at some point.

When I asked her whether she had ever considered why she was so "accident prone," she looked at me blankly and said: *I am not sure what you are asking. I am just a very unlucky person. The worst things always happen to me.* It was quite obvious that she was not seeing what I was seeing and if I had pushed the issue, she would stop talking to me. Then, out of the blue, her son announced that he was going to move in with his girlfriend who lived in a city a few hours away. Two days later, the mother had another accident. This time she ended up with a whiplash and was told to stay at home and rest for at least three weeks. Of course, any plans of her son moving had to be put on hold. Her children were quite worried about her condition, as she was in a lot of pain. I was concerned myself. It was painful to watch. I was willing to bet that by the time those three weeks had passed, she would not be necessarily getting better, and unfortunately, I was right.

She was getting far too much attention from her kids to allow herself to heal. Three weeks later, she was insisting that she was still in a lot of pain and unable to perform certain tasks, such as housework. What was interesting was that her doctor recommended a number of strategies to improve her situation, including physiotherapy and chiropractic treatments, but after a couple of appointments, she would decide that it was not working for her and refused to continue. She actually ended up being officially classified as disabled. Under the circumstances, her children had to take turns to make sure that she got the help she needed with those everyday activities she was no longer able to do. This went on for several months.

The weather then started getting better, and as she loved her gardening, she was now in conflict. All of this was subconscious, of course. On the one hand, the benefit of maintaining this injury meant she was getting attention from her children that she craved so much, as well as disability benefits. However, it also meant she was unable to work in the garden, and that was making her more and more unhappy. She got cornered by her subconscious mind. In the end, what she was getting out of living with the chronic injury and pain turned out to hold more power.

I ended up moving to a different part for the country, and we lost contact, but my guess is that she would have found the way to keep her children close, regardless of the cost to her and to them. Such is the power of the subconscious mind and secondary gain.

In this chapter, we are going to focus on building self-awareness, as this is critical to your overall success with the healing process. This is because awareness is critical to creating any lasting change. In fact, you are going to be expanding your awareness the entire time you are engaging with this book, but in this section, I will introduce you to some of the most powerful awareness building tools that I use. We will start with understanding emotional toxicity and assessing where you are on the emotional toxicity spectrum. Even though chronic stress is often mentioned as one of the key contributing factors to chronic illness, the approach to addressing it is mostly superficial.

Not many practitioners have adequate understanding or skills when it comes to properly addressing the psycho-energetic root causes of ill health, which go very far beyond the day-to-day stress, such as financial problems or misbehaving children. I do appreciate that people cannot be trained in everything under the sun, and I am not necessarily expecting practitioners to be able to help their clients to fully address these psycho-energetic factors. The reality is that this is quite a complex area of work. What I am expecting, however, is more awareness from practitioners that just telling their clients to do some meditation to manage their stress is doing people a massive disservice.

This is because for most people with chronic health issues, "doing some meditation" is simply not enough, as they are pretty much always highly emotionally toxic. So even when they follow this inadequate prescription, they will feel like they are failing to handle the matter, or that there is something wrong them. It is important to at least let people know that their state of health is a product of many years of energetic imbalances and nervous system dysregulation resulting from different traumas (including attachment and intergenerational trauma), as well as social engineering. That way, when they struggle to manage their emotional toxicity with meditation, they do not feel like failures but instead have a proper appreciation that we are dealing with energetic, neurological and emotional complexity here.

Emotional Symptoms

So that you can have a full appreciation of the fact that this work is about much more than your day-to-day stress, below is a list of some most common emotional toxicity symptoms. Please keep in mind these become toxic when experienced chronically:

- poor self-worth/poor self-esteem
- negative self-talk
- feeling undeserving
- guilt
- shame
- feeling anxious or worried
- fears (e.g., fear of rejection/criticism, fear of failure, fear of losing control, fear of death/illness, etc.)
- feeling sadness or grief
- feeling defensive
- feeling jealous/envious
- feeling anger, frustration or rage
- over-analyzing or over-thinking
- feeling overwhelmed
- feeling negative
- not being able to think clearly
- experiencing ruminating thoughts
- being critical of others or yourself
- feeling irritable
- feeling depressed/apathetic
- feeling victimized
- feeling unsure of yourself and/or questioning your decisions
- feeling alienated
- being in a toxic relationship

- being a doormat
- mental rehearsals
- not being able to forgive others or yourself
- anything that stops your mind from being silent and stops you from experiencing inner peace

But all these are just SYMPTOMS and people with chronic health issues who are serious about their recovery must identify and deal with the root causes of these symptoms!

Why? Because:

EMOTIONAL TOXICITY = CHRONIC STRESS = NERVOUS SYSTEM DYSREGULATION AND POOR VAGAL TONE = YOU CANNOT HEAL

We will talk about the mechanisms of this in more detail in the next chapter, but for now, remember that you can only heal when you spend enough time in the rest-digest-detoxify-heal response. You are not able to heal if you spend most of your time in survival states of fight, flight, or freeze, which many people do. In addition, studies have shown that chronic cortisol exposure associated with chronic stress impacts epigenetic processes and increases your risk of experiencing not only physical but also psychological issues in the long run.

Key Root Causes of Emotional Toxicity Symptoms

On the level of mind and neurology: stress in utero, birth trauma, intergenerational trauma, early life exposure to stress, childhood trauma (attachment issues, one-off traumas as well as repetitive traumas), as well as early conditioning (social engineering) are the main root causes of emotional toxicity. These affect our personality traits, our value and belief systems, and our identity and self-worth. They contribute to internal conflicts and even what people will attract. As we then progress through life, we experience other traumas and everyday challenges that further contribute to our nervous system imbalance and our overall level of emotional toxicity. Believe it or not, this is just on the mind level. In addition to that, any disturbances we have in our biofield will feed into this. If we are imbalanced energetically, and most people with chronic health issues are, this can contribute to internal conflicts, can attract traumas and toxic relationships, and can contribute to a person experiencing chronic fears, anxieties, and so on.

When you address your root causes of emotional toxicity, you are able to quiet your mind, which means you will be able to spend more time in the parasympathetic rest-digest-detoxify-heal response. This, in turn, means less inflammation, less tissue destruction, more energy, and more effective healing! Before you move on, please take my Emotional Toxicity Questionnaire, which you can find in the Additional Resources in order to assess where you currently are on the emotional toxicity spectrum.

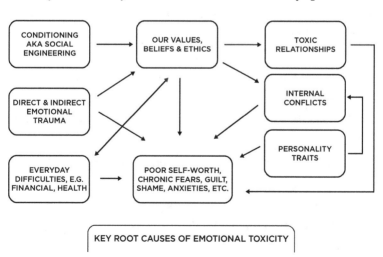

89

Secondary Gain

Everybody who has ever studied the mind of people with chronic illness will tell you that most people with long-term symptoms or illness have a SUBCONSCIOUS *resistance to health*. This is called secondary gain, which can be defined as: *a benefit realized by not recovering from a mental or physical dysfunction*. You may be feeling yourself getting irritated right now, thinking: *How dare you tell me I have resistance to health? That is stupid. Of course I want to be healthy. Is this not why I am reading this book?*

Let me clarify. I did say subconscious, right? So do I believe that you consciously want to be healthy? Absolutely. 100 percent. Otherwise, you would not be reading this book. However, remember what we said about the conscious and the subconscious mind, and how if there is no agreement between them, it is the subconscious that is going to come out on top? The subconscious is automatic, it is faster, and 95 percent of the time it dominates your life. So when we have somebody who says they want to heal and their subconscious is fully on board with that idea, what do you think happens? They heal. It is as simple as that.

Why? Because there is nothing within their mind to oppose or sabotage the healing process, so the signals the mind is sending to the body are conducive to healing. Again, for this to be the case, the subconscious must be programed for healing and the person must believe they deserve to be healthy, which means the person feels worthy. When these boxes are checked, healing is usually a natural progression. The only exception to this rule is if there is something purely at the biofield level that is obstructing the healing, or there is some external factor that is powerful enough to cause damage even after we have tidied the mind up, e.g., or a cell phone tower right outside your bedroom. But even when faced with those external factors, we stand much more of a chance if the brain, the nervous system, and the biofield are in good shape.

Let me give you a real-life example. I had a long-term gastritis, which is inflammation of the stomach lining. I was not able to shift it for several years. I analyzed my beliefs to the n-th degree. I knew it was not a self-worth issue either, and no amount of herbs or supplements, or even using bioresonance technology designed to assess and treat misalignments within the biofield, was making it go away. It would go through a cycle of it subsiding and returning over and over. I eventually concluded it was an energetic issue and even suspected that geopathic burden (resulting from a disrupted electromagnetic field of the Earth) was to blame. We did have a geopathic stress issue at the house we lived in at the time. But then we moved, and this was no longer an issue. I can measure geopathic stress with a bioresonance device I have, so that is how I know. My problem however, persisted. I was still convinced the issue was energetic so I started digging around and exploring family karma and family programs. I came to realize that this issue originated a few months after my grandmother had died. My grandma was a big part of my life and my upbringing. I have already shared with you that my grandmother's daughter died from a vaccine injury and because of this my grandma carried an enormous amount of guilt all her life. My grandma also had a lot of anger, mainly with herself, which she held onto until she died. For decades my grandma was on medication for gastritis and gastroduodenitis. Her stomach area was where she stored her guilt, her anger, and also her grief in the body. She never dealt with the trauma of losing her child, and her stomach problems in my opinion were 100 percent linked to that.

I realized that soon after my grandma had died, my stomach started giving me issues. I had a Reiki session, and it was confirmed that I was storing a lot of anger and grief in that area of my body. I realized that these emotions were not mine. I was so close to my grandma that somehow I inherited her grief and her anger too! I had some of my own anger to work through, but not all of it was mine. The grief was not mine either. When I realized that, I started releasing this emotional charge from my body. I talked to my grandma and said: *Grandma, I love you but I cannot carry this for you. Please take it back. Otherwise, it will end up killing me and I know you do not want me to be harmed by this.* I was not being melodramatic. Unresolved gastritis usually leads to ulcers, and stomach ulcers have been linked to stomach cancer, so it was important to resolve this once and for all. After quite a number of years of chasing my tail with this issue, it was this epiphany, and releasing the pent-up energy, that was not even mine, that got my stomach to start to heal properly. So it is true that the subconscious resistance to healing is not the ultimate barrier 100 percent of the time, but 90 percent of the time there is some form of block at the subconscious level, and this must be addressed.

So what could be somebody's secondary gain? Here are some examples:

- getting attention, nurturance or sympathy
- avoiding responsibility
- withdrawal or not wanting to deal with the world (due to loss, money issues, etc.)
- feeling emotionally or physically safer with the illness
- using illness as an excuse for lack of success

- using illness as punishment (for others or self)
- not feeling deserving of health
- fear of change or fear of the unknown (familiarity, however uncomfortable, is safer)
- fear of commitment
- learning (experiencing this problem helps the person learn more about themselves, others, the illness, etc.)
- feeling special
- illness has become the person's identity (or part of their identity) and they do not want to give up part of themselves
- illness is a barometer that keeps somebody in line (letting them know they are too stressed, that their emotions are out of balance, their boundaries are not being respected, etc.)
- fear of freedom
- fear of success
- being held back so that the person does not rush into things that may hurt them
- controlling other people's behavior
- acting in accordance with false scripts (e.g., my father/mother had this illness, so I have to have it too to prove my "hypothesis" was right)
- receiving money, e.g., benefits.

There is also enmeshment. This is when somebody is stuck in a codependent relationship where the boundary between one person ends and their partner begins is fuzzy and not clearly defined. The relationship is the secondary gain here because of this idea that it is better to be miserable in a relationship than have no relationship. So the relationship might be a massive contributing factor to the illness, in this case, and, at the same time, the reason why somebody will be stuck and unable to get better, which makes it a real trap.

Uncovering Your Secondary Gain

So I want you to ask yourself the following questions now and answer with the first thing that comes to mind. Do not overthink this because then you are engaging your conscious analytical mind and you want the answers to come from your subconscious. Also, be mindful of any bodily sensations or emotional responses you may have as you are doing this exercise.

- What is my secondary gain?
- How am I benefiting from keeping myself in this state? What am I getting out of it?
- What purpose is this health issue serving? What is its job?
- If I didn't have this problem, what would I have to do that I don't have to do at the moment? What am I seeking to avoid? What am I resisting?
- If I lose this health problem, what else will I lose with it?
- In what way is my health issue an attempt to survive or to be safe?
- What are my symptoms saying to me? If my body could speak, what would it say?
- If my physical condition was a negative emotion, what would it be?
- How is my body a reflection of my current life?
- How is my body reflecting my past?
- When will I have suffered enough?

Hopefully, you have now taken the first step to understanding what is blocking you from healing. If you were not able to get any answers, that is fine too. Please, do not fret about it.

94

You will have plenty of other opportunities to uncover whatever you need to uncover. You are not necessarily going to be able to identify your secondary gain right away. You may have to build more awareness or take off some of those outer emotional layers first. Let that be OK. If you have got some answers from doing this exercise but you have no idea what any of it means, that is great. Write all of it down. There will come a point when you will have that "aha" moment.

Now, let us approach this slightly differently. Here is a set of statements. Again, do not overthink this and watch out for any bodily sensations or emotional responses you may have that let you know if a given statement feels true or false to you.

- My health problem helps me attract sympathy, attention, nurturing and/or social connection.
- My health problem makes me feel special.
- My health problem helps me control and dominate the behavior of others.
- My health problem helps me punish myself for real and imagined sins.
- My health problem helps me punish others.
- My health problem helps me avoid responsibility.
- My health problem helps me avoid having to deal with the world.
- My health problem helps me feel safe.
- My health problem gives me an excuse for not achieving or meeting other people's expectations of me.
- My health problem gives me an excuse not to change.
- My health problem gives me an excuse for when I feel/ look foolish (*Can't help it. It is because I have this problem.*)
- My health problem gives me an opportunity to learn and experience.

95

- My health problem is my barometer that lets me know that I am out of balance.
- My health problem is part of who I am. I would be lost without it.
- My health problem holds me back so that I do not rush into things that may harm me.
- My health problem ensures I am in a relationship.
- My health problem is genetic. I have it because it runs in the family.
- My health problem results in me receiving financial benefits.

So perhaps you have just confirmed what you have already discovered previously, or maybe you have just realized what is blocking you from healing. If these exercises have helped you uncover something new, that is brilliant. If you are still not sure what you secondary gain might be, please be patient. The answers will come.

Identifying Your Attachment Adaptations

If you have not previously looked into attachment styles, you will hopefully find this information quite enlightening. Recognizing your attachment style is, in my opinion, one of the key aspects of building self-awareness. This will really help you understand why you currently think, feel, and behave the way you do. The information in this section is based on the work of John Bowlby, Mary Ainsworth, and Diane Poole Heller.

When faced with a threat, our bodies generate various forms of survival energy. When the fight-or-flight response kicks in, we can run, pounce, attack, destroy, etc. These are normal responses if we are being threatened. The problem is when we get stuck in this charged state for too long. Our circuits get fried, so to speak, and we dissociate. So those same life-saving responses that allow us to escape a threat or fight it off can stay trapped in our bodies and get caught on a feedback loop. This is a destructive cycle because if our bodies are stuck in survival mode, everything is interpreted as a threat, which affects how we relate to others and ourselves.

As we have already briefly mentioned, when we are born, we have many needs—not just physical but also neurological and emotional. If those are not adequately met, that compromises our sense of safety and negatively impacts our development. As babies, we need skin-to-skin contact, cuddles, and kisses to let us know we are safe, loved, and protected. Otherwise, our nervous system has a neurological deficiency, which, in turn, causes all sorts of trust and attachment issues. Remember that unless we feel 100 percent safe, we enter one of the survival states. When the nervous system responds as if there is a threat, our brain is focused on surviving and not on self-awareness and connecting to others. If this turns chronic, this also is one of the key contributing factors to ill health.

The problem is that not many people grow up feeling safe, loved, and protected, not necessarily because the parents are narcissists or psychopaths, although that also happens, but because the caregivers may have their own attachment issues, unresolved trauma, unhelpful beliefs, not to mention pressures of everyday life. So, unfortunately, not many babies have a consistent enough environment of protection, love, care, positive physical connection, awareness, and responsiveness.

Safety is not just critical in childhood, of course. It is also important in adulthood. Our brain is highly attuned to this. We know right away when we have a connection with somebody and when we do not, and safety is an important aspect of that. Overall, we do much better physically and emotionally when we have a perception of being understood, seen, heard, and felt. However, that is not the case in many relationships because of insecure attachment.

Before we proceed to discussing attachment patterns, remember not to give yourself a hard time about your current attachment style. You have developed it because that was the way your nervous system knew how to keep you safe. It is an adaptation and it can definitely be altered. Again, as you continue to read, and determine that you identify with a particular attachment adaptation, accept where you are at this time and set an intention to move towards secure attachment.

Secure Attachment

Secure people grew up with love, support and protection. Their needs where consistently met. Secure attachment is how we are designed to operate in the world. Even if it feels like a distant dream to you right now, believe me that your secure attachment is there waiting for you to dust it off and reconnect with it. Even if we fall out of it at times, it is there for us to return to. As we become more secure, we are more receptive, less reactive, more emotionally available, more connected, and, of course, healthier. Plus, we become better parents and better partners for others and can help our loved ones step into secure attachment too.

Developing a secure attachment in childhood doesn't necessarily mean always getting what we want. It is not about that.

However, just feeding and clothing a child is not enough to produce a secure attachment either. That emotional nurturing piece is key. Ed Tronick, a developmental psychologist, shows through his research that if we feel secure for about 30 percent of the time in childhood, we are likely to attach securely. For this to be the case, our safety needs to be somebody's priority, our environment needs to be stable and consistent, and our needs must be taken care of. But the key takeaway here is that parents do not have to get it right 100 percent of the time. Just as well really, because that would not be achievable for any parent, no matter how loving and caring they are. Remember that whether a child feels their needs are met or not has nothing to do with objective reality and everything to do with how this child internalizes what goes on around them. So expecting any parent to be able to work that out accurately 100 percent of the time is completely unrealistic. Even a third of the time is a stretch, but at least that is more achievable.

Just to clarify, being protected does not mean being smothered and micromanaged. We still need our independence and autonomy as children. As Diane Poole Heller says: *For secure attachment the balance and flow between being together and being apart must be just right.* It is also key that a child can express themselves in the way they want and still be accepted. The moment the child feels they need to mold themselves into something they are not, because a caregiver expects them to act or feel differently, we have a problem. Firstly, this introduces stress, which starts to negatively condition the nervous system. But even more importantly, the child gets this idea: *I am not OK as I am. I must be somebody else to be accepted and loved.* This is particularly problematic for children, as this is the beginning of the erosion of this child's identity, which is at the core of people's ill health. It also is important that the child's environment is reasonably relaxed, without constant tension, anger, fear, etc. Small children take everything at face value and process the world around them through their feelings. If they pick up on fear in their environment, it will make them feel fearful. This, again, will make them feel unsafe, and they will come to the same conclusion: *I am not OK.*

Adults with secure attachment styles:

- find it easy to connect to others and be relaxed around them, have no problems being affectionate and intimate, and expect relationships to go well

- transition effortlessly between alone time and time with others

- apologize easily and work to find win-win solutions to any conflicts that arise

- believe that people are basically good at heart

- find it easy to ask for support and to have their own needs met and are receptive to the needs of the people they are close to

- look forward to spending time with their partner and friends and stay present and free from distractions when doing so

- respect others' needs for privacy and set healthy boundaries

- are aware enough to recognize when things are not working in a relationship and leave knowing there are other great options for fulfilling relationships.

As you read on, be aware that the remaining attachment styles (Avoidant, Ambivalent, Disorganized) are adaptations, due to challenging childhood circumstances and the child's internal responses to their external environment. **A person can exhibit a mix of styles depending on circumstances.** For example, you could become disorganized under a particular type of stress only. It is about finding your dominant pattern. The aim is to shift back into secure attachment.

As we already said, we develop these different attachment adaptations in order to ensure our survival when we are children. Once the nervous system is developed and conditioned to run those patterns, they will persist until we become aware of them and take active steps to change them. If your dominant style were already strongly secure, you would likely not be reading this book as you would not have that much of a need for it. Unless of course, you are reading it to help others. The majority of challenges we are trying to address with this method are associated with insecure attachment. Most people would reach for a book like this because they recognize that certain aspects of their lives are not how they want them to be and because they want to change them. So accept where you are for now. Whatever it is, let that be OK.

Avoidant Attachment Style

Avoidant attachment style develops when a child is left alone for extended periods of time, when they are ignored or neglected, or when there is any form of incongruence, such as expressive dissonance, when facial expression does not match the caregiver's emotional state. It may be that caregivers are not present, or they might be physically present but emotionally unavailable, or they may be present only when they are trying to teach the child something. Avoidant attachment will develop if touch is mostly absent, when even though people are around, there is lack of appropriate physical contact.

The child needs the contact, but since it is not forthcoming, they get used to not having it, and this becomes their "normal." That causes the child to be disconnected, but since this is what they are accustomed to, that is what feels safe. This, by the way, does not stop them from feeling rejected, unlovable, and abandoned deep inside. Just because they have found the way to survive and stay safe does not mean they feel good about themselves or feel happy. Remember that children tend to blame themselves for their caregivers' shortcomings or anything that is not right in their environment. Again, for this adaptation to develop, caregivers do not have to be narcissistic or sociopathic, but, of course, the situation is even more serious when there is emotional and/or physical neglect.

Avoidants might appear aloof and as though they do not need anybody, but this is nothing more than fear of being vulnerable with others. They view it as a big risk. People do not feel safe to them. They might even consciously believe relationships have nothing to offer them, but they subconsciously crave connection. This results in emotional turmoil. We all want connection, even if some people claim they do not need it. Avoidants can be also perceived as detached, insensitive, cold, and standoffish. This comes from growing up feeling isolated.

Avoidants, much like people with an ambivalent and disorganized attachment styles, have a lot of self-loathing. This because they spent their early years feeling: *I am not OK. There is something inherently wrong with me.* It can feel normal for Avoidants to dissociate, and it is a useful strategy when the stress of connecting to others starts to overwhelm them. They often distract with the Internet, games, and TV. Even meditating can be a form of avoidance if it becomes an excuse to be on their own. Even though these activities can make them feel calmer, they make them feel less connected.

Adults with avoidant attachment style:

- find close relationships challenging, which often means frequently changing partners, as they find closeness uncomfortable and feel suffocated by it

- find it difficult to relax or be intimate with their partners and tend to avoid close physical contact and eye contact

- find it difficult to confide in others, ask for help, or to ask for what they need

- prefer to work alone and engage in solo activities rather than be with others, and their work is more important than their personal relationships (they tend to be task-focused, efficient, and productive)

- find people who are emotional, effusive, use "too many words" to describe their experiences, or lack self-sufficiency to be off-putting

- tend to be more left-brain dominant: more factual, analytical, and logical, which when too extreme may mean lack of emotional warmth, being out of touch with their intuition, and lack of interpersonal skills

- prefer relationships with animals, plants, or objects over relationships with people, as that feels safer to them

- tend to be dismissive of their past and may even portray their childhood in a positive light because they disconnected from the past and are not aware that their emotional needs were not met

- tend to feel an initial wave of relief when ending a relationship, which tends to be followed by polar opposite feelings like depression or despair

- feel more available and connected to their previous partners when the pressure of the relationship is off

- feel there is a perfect someone out there who they have not met yet and that it is easier to chase that fantasy than enjoy and commit to the person they are actually with.

Avoidants need time to transition between being on their own and reconnecting with others. Allowing them that time can do a lot for the relationship. If they are going to become more secure, it is important for them to learn to give and receive help. Practicing being more generous and comfortable with physical gestures and closeness is also a step towards a more secure attachment. If you believe this may be your dominant attachment style, one thing you can do right away is to connect with your loved one or a friend by participating in a joint activity that you will give 100 percent of your attention to. If you feel uncomfortable when you do this and, you acknowledge what you are feeling, you give yourself permission to feel it deeply (I recommend expressing what you are feeling out loud), and watch the feeling dissipate. The feeling will only persist if you resist it. You can then carry on with the activity.

Ambivalent Attachment Style

Ambivalent or anxious attachment develops when a child has a lot of anxiety about having their needs met or being loved or lovable. Ambivalents usually were lucky enough to receive affection from their primary caregivers. The problem was that the affection was not consistent or predictable enough, due to poor awareness, unresolved trauma, etc. They never knew when their caregivers may withdraw their affection or pull the rug from under their feet in one way or another. When children experience inconsistent or unreliable care, it is confusing, which causes anxiety. That teaches them that they cannot reliably expect positive connections with others. Because they did not experience consistent enough parental receptivity, they struggle to self-regulate later in life and have to rely on others to fulfil that original need that was never met when they were children. This is why they tend to look to others to put them at ease or calm down their overactive nervous system. Whilst Avoidants get triggered by connection, Ambivalents experience stress on loss of contact.

Adults with ambivalent attachment style:

- struggle to be alone, as that tends to make them feel abandoned, anxious, hurt, sad, or angry

- find it difficult to say *no* to others and set healthy boundaries

- tend to be over-focused on others, and neglect themselves and their own needs

- find relationships to be unpredictable and erratic

- tend to apologize for things they have not done when they are scared of upsetting or losing their partner

- find themselves yearning for people who feel unavailable to them

- often second-guess themselves and lack confidence

- can be needy, clingy, oversensitive, controlling, jealous, obsessive, high-maintenance, or highly strung and need others to calm them down, as they find it difficult to self-soothe

- feel like they give more than they receive in relationships, which makes them feel resentful towards the other person

- find it difficult to recognize when their partner expresses love and appreciation, tend to overlook or dismiss caring behaviors from others

- feel they can easily attune to others' feelings, wants, and needs and tend to be right-brain dominant

- often find themselves living in the past, not able to forgive or forget old injuries

- want connection yet feel afraid of losing whatever relationship they are in

- can be hypervigilant and overreact to any perceived hint of abandonment, anticipating the abandonment before anything actually happens in the relationship

- feel upset or pick fights whenever the partner has to be away from them.

Ambivalents are in near-constant fight-or-flight, as they always feel threatened and expect to be abandoned. Often, they suffer from chronic illness, which is their cry for attention and affection. This could also be punishment, as deep inside they believe they are not deserving. They can be extreme in their behavior and push people away so their fear is realized. This, in turn, confirms their original hypothesis that they are not lovable and that people will only hurt them and let them down. So again, we are dealing with self-loathing here. This constant seeking for others to soothe them stems from poor self-worth and lack of connection with themselves. They are a bottomless bucket. Because the bottom of the bucket (self-love) is missing, no matter how much affection other people put into their bucket, it falls right out.

Ambivalents, when consistently reassured, will eventually learn to trust the relationship, but, of course, self-love is key to work on. Ambivalents dismiss caring behaviors and deny things are good because admitting that a relationship is going well comes with fear of losing it. They need to focus on caring behaviors for long enough for the nervous system to register the safety that comes with such behaviors. If you recognize this adaptation as your dominant pattern, you can start doing small things to help you soothe your nervous system right away, such as wrapping yourself in a blanket, self-massage, or anything else that makes you feel soothed.

Disorganized Attachment Style

Disorganized attachment is much less studied, but it stems from excessive fear in our original attachment relationship. Caregivers may have been dangerous or threatening to the child, or living in fear themselves, had unresolved trauma, or may have been dissociated. Birth trauma, overwhelming events, or medical procedures that interrupt the parent-child connection early on can contribute. Other possible factors include: poverty, starvation, illness, addictions, and caregivers who shift states abruptly, giving the child confusing messages.

In the end, the child's conclusion is that relationships are dangerous.

When a child is stressed, they naturally seek comfort and protection from their caregivers but if the caregivers themselves are the threat, the child will get stuck in the fear response. That makes them emotionally dysregulated or completely dissociated. They suffer from psychological and physical confusion. When the caregivers are scared, they cannot regulate their own distress so they cannot calm the child. This results in the child being in fight-or flight, or shutdown (freeze), most of the time. Their resilience is limited at that age, so any emotion can become overwhelming and lead to the child acting out. They are then punished, which makes everything worse. This may contribute to addictions, psychiatric conditions, personality disorders, violence, or even criminal behaviors.

At the very least, they tend to misread others, get defensive, aggressive, controlling, and struggle to form meaningful connections they so badly need for healing. People with this attachment style suffer from ongoing sense of failure and intense self-loathing. They may go towards danger because it is their "normal." Paradoxically, putting themselves in life-threatening situations has a certain familiarity to it. They learn to ignore threats because constantly feeling threatened made them lose the ability to tell danger from safety. Disorganized attachment is a mixture of an avoidant and ambivalent attachment with the addition of intense fear due to the ever-present threat. Some people with this attachment style are more avoidant, others more anxious and panicky. There are also those who swing back and forth and get diagnosed with disorders such a bipolar.

Adults with disorganized attachment style:

- perceive intimate relationships as dangerous

- may become frozen or immobile in relationship with others, particularly when they feel blocked or trapped, and may experience an inexplicable fear when they reach a certain level of intimacy

- tend to have an exaggerated startle response when people approach them unexpectedly

- tend to be controlling

- often expect that the worst will happen in relationships and struggle to feel safe with their partner, even when they know the other person is trustworthy

- often disconnect, dissociate, or become confused in relationships and fear that close relationships may trigger dysregulation that is difficult to manage

- have a difficult time remembering significant events, past relationships, or how they made them feel

- often experience sudden and unpredictable shifts of state (for example, switching from joy and happiness to fear and anger)

- when triggered, they become stressed or confused by complicated instructions and arrangements

- can feel set up to fail and unable to solve problems

- long to connect with others while, at the same time, wanting to get away from them.

Disorganized attachment style is associated with the freeze response. In freeze state the body reduces the intake of oxygen, so deep slow breathing is very beneficial to start reconditioning the nervous system as is moving the body around. Yoga, qigong, and tai chi can be particularly helpful. These strategies will, of course, benefit you greatly whatever your attachment style is at this time.

To summarize, early experiences prime us for threat or safety, but either way we have neuroplasticity to fall back on. This means we can heal whatever is making us insecure and make the secure traits more dominant, as we are actually biologically programmed for secure attachment. Even though it is true that our primal brain is always on the lookout for threats, our nervous system is capable of more than just focusing on basic survival. This why with the right approach and tools we can make ourselves feel more secure and resilient. Before you move on to the next section, close your eyes and think who in your life helps you feel safe and relaxed. Maybe it is a person, maybe a pet. Connect with them in your mind and notice what sensations and emotions that produces for you. Where do you feel those in your body? Just spend a few minutes enjoying these feelings and the healing effect this has on your nervous system.

What Is Your Enneagram Type?

Understanding attachment styles is one way of getting to know yourself and having awareness of where some of your adaptive behaviors originated from. There are many other tools that can help you get to know yourself and your responses better. In this category, I include personality profiling tools, of which there are quite a few. Some are better than others. One my favorites, which I encourage you to explore in more detail, is the Enneagram. The reason why I like this one so much is that it shows you where you currently are but it also shows you your growth path. Each type is a spectrum, and you aim to evolve along that spectrum.

The Enneagram is a discovery developed through observation. It is not a creation. It is a personality pattern typing system that helps you understand yourself and others. Carl Gustav Jung, a Swiss psychiatrist and psychoanalyst, was one of the first people who observed that there are only so many patterns of behavior observed in humans, even though we are all unique beings. The Enneagram essentially focuses on nine reasons WHY we behave the way we do. So we have nine types within which there are levels of growth expression. We aim to grow, or evolve, to our highest expression. There are many Enneagram teachers. Personally, I resonate the most with the approach presented by an Enneagram coach, Colleen-Joy Page. If you want to, you can watch my interview with Colleen-Joy, which can be found in the Additional Resources.

What you need to be aware of is that even the best online Enneagram tests are only 50 to 60 percent accurate. This is because those questionnaires struggle to capture WHY you behave the way you do, which forms the basis of this personality profiling tool. I encourage you to read as many descriptions as you can find of the different types to really confirm which type you are. I will be giving you a very brief summary of each type here to get you started. When you are going through the types, you will likely identify with more than one type to begin with, but one should dominate. If you are unsure, you will need to do more reading around this, and again, I encourage you to watch the video I am sharing. Also, the more self-awareness you build, the clearer you will be on your dominant type.

It is important that you are honest with yourself. In order to improve and evolve, you need to know where you are right now and be acceptant of wherever that is. It is my opinion that there is no point sugar-coating this as that is not helping you grow. Each of the types has its positive and negative aspects. The reality is that people who have not done much, or any, self-development work are more likely to be at the lower end of expression of their respective type. That is why what we are doing with this method is often described as shadow work, and in order to transmute your shadow you need to see it first. Ultimately, to be quite blunt, until you are ready to face your current shortcomings and call yourself on your own nonsense, it is just words on paper, i.e. meaningless. So let's do this, shall we?

Enneagram – Type 1

They resist everything that is below par, not perfect, immoral, that does not follow the rules, etc. Under stress, they go to anger. This can be mild irritation, grumpiness, or full-blown hysterical rage. Type 1 is always trying to be "good," which means that they try to manage their anger and contain it. They are principled, purposeful, and self-controlled. They have a fierce inner critic that is always looking to be perfect. They are also critical towards others. They teach or instruct others how to be "good." They want to improve things all the time. They think in terms of right or wrong, nothing in the middle. Something cannot be 70 percent right. It is either right or wrong. Rules are important to them. They have high standards and high morals. They use words such as *should* and *must* a lot. At their stress point, they tend to display the worst characteristics of type 4 on the Enneagram. This means theatrical anger. What they need to do in order to evolve within their type is to encourage themselves to move towards their polarity (type 7), which means being free-spirited, youthful, spontaneous, and fun. When they can access these characteristics, they feel freer and more relaxed. They start to use their intuitive instincts, and this softens them.

Enneagram – Type 2

Type 2 wants to be seen as a giving and generous person. It is particularly important for them to feel needed, loved, and appreciated. They are, therefore, trying to be helpful and caring, and the more helpful they feel, the more worthy they feel. They can get resentful if they are not appreciated. If their sense of worth is really low, they might exaggerate some of their qualities in order to be seen as helpful (people-pleasing). They can be smothering and possessive because they really value connections and relationships above all else. Always aware of what other people need, they put a lot of effort into being nice. They are proud to be an ideal friend, partner, lover, work colleague, etc. At their stress point, when they are at their lowest, they tend to take on some of the characteristics of type 8. This is when they feel their giving has not been appreciated and their resentment comes out as anger. At their best, they take on the positive characteristics of type 4. That is when they learn to notice their own feelings, their own needs, and they are able to look after themselves without guilt. They discover self-love, which enables them to give even more. Because they are now receptive to their own needs, they are able to really share from their heart.

Enneagram – Type 3

Type 3 wants to be seen as *the best*. They are success-oriented, driven, adaptive, and pragmatic. Goals are very important to them. For them failure triggers a sense of low worth. They are invested in striving, achieving, and winning. They are a *yes* person because saying *no* might imply that they cannot do it. It is only as they evolve within their type that they learn to say *no*. They can be quite charming. They know how to work a relationship or a room. They want to do everything quicker, easier, and in the most efficient way. There is so much to do and very little time to do it. They like to-do lists. They tend to expect people in their life to also be striving and they do not have much tolerance for "losers". They are quite focused on their own needs, own wants, and own vision. They can suffer from a bit of vanity. At their stress point, they tend display some of the worst characteristics of type 9. This means that they procrastinate and avoid. Sometimes, when they have taken on too much, the pressure comes, and they realize that they might fail to impress and deliver. When they access the best characteristics of type 6, which is their polarity, they discover deep meaning of success. When they choose service to other people in order to succeed, they are now making a difference and changing lives, instead of winning for the sake of winning. Now they motivate and inspire others.

Enneagram – Type 4

Type 4 is the sensitive and expressive type. They want to be seen as unique and until they know their own worth, they are going to exaggerate their uniqueness in order to validate their worth. At their stress point, they take on the worst characteristics of type 2. They become needy, clingy, and may also look for people to save that are more broken than they are. At their worst, their emotions become theatrical. They become dramatic, self-absorbed, and temperamental. It is all about them and what they

114

want. Their real emotions are always safely hidden but on the surface, it can be a storm of moodiness and extreme emotions. They tend to move through life looking at things differently. They do not like the Enneagram because they do not want to be put in a box. Sometimes they feel like an outsider looking into the world, believing other people have it better than they do. If their wounds help them to be seen as unique, they cling to their wounds. They want to stay broken in order to attract attention and to feel worthy. If life is ordinary, they do not feel alive. They can suffer from melancholy. At their best, they access the most desirable characteristics of type 1. They realize that feelings are not facts and that they are already unique, which makes them feel secure. They become healthy and functional, channeling their sensitivity and emotions appropriately.

Enneagram – Type 5

Type 5 is dominated by their mind. You can describe them as "intensely cerebral." Thinking is their primary source of decision-making. They value their mind because their mind is a place of escaping and coping with their fear. They use thinking to help them feel safe, to manage their fear, and to channel it into something constructive. When they want to understand something, they want to understand it fully. They separate themselves from people and they keep themselves at a distance. They can be secretive and isolate themselves. It is natural for them to prefer to observe rather than engage. They want to understand first. When they finally do understand, then they will feel safe enough to jump in and engage with life. People might experience them as cold and non-expressive. In reality, they are checking to see whether they can trust people before they connect, which is always on the mind level. At their worst, some of the destructive characteristics of type 7 show up in them, and their mind becomes chaotic. When they access the best characteristics of their opposite, which is type 8, they find courage and they learn to channel their mind and bring their knowledge into the real world. They grow in confidence. They discover that their wisdom and knowledge is worth sharing. Their growth is to learn to not just observe but to apply practically. They have a lot to offer others when they learn to connect with people without fear.

Enneagram – Type 6

Type 6 is security oriented. They are always questioning, *what-if-ing*, planning, controlling, and thinking. Their decision making is very strongly directed by their mind and by their anxiety or fear. They are always looking for ways to be safe and secure. Their mind will run at thousand miles per hour to find safety in something. They ask many questions to help alleviate their anxiety. Belonging, loyalty, and responsibility are very important to them. At their lowest point, they worry a lot. Even when things are going well, they might worry about the fact that they are going well. They are very discerning, which helps them work out who they can trust. They want to trust but they find it challenging. When they are feeling insecure, they can be cold and separate. When they are stressed, they go to the worst characteristics of type 3, pretending to be confident when they are not. They then have the tendency to manipulate in order to belong. When they go to their polarity, which is type 9, they finally learn to relax in their skin and slow down. They learn to just be, and they learn the difference between thinking and knowing. When they learn to trust their knowing, they settle and find support and safety within themselves. This alleviates their fear. They then contribute to life, which is their highest aspiration.

Enneagram – Type 7

Type 7 is always trying to have fun in order to not face their fear and anxiety. Fun makes them feel safe. They might not appear to be an anxious person at all. In fact, they may create an impression of being brave because they tend to be adrenaline junkies. They believe it is okay for them to take risks as long as they are having fun. However, at their lowest, this side of them is a result of their anxiety. They can be distracted, unfocused, and scattered, moving from one idea to another. They do not want to do the same thing again and again. That would be boring, and boredom makes them feel anxious. They value freedom and want to do what they want when they want to. Sitting still is difficult for them. They can push themselves to the point of collapse because they have a fear of missing out. They love life, like to keep busy and explore, but it is actually difficult for them to be present in the now moment until they have evolved within their type. People experience them as happy, as they tend to be very positive, even when very bad things happen. However, at their stress point, they tend to go drop into the worst characteristics of type 1. They suddenly start being incredibly critical, pedantic, and quite angry and hard on themselves. Fortunately, they do not like to stay there long. Ideally, they need to access the best characteristics of type 5, when they learn to sit still. Then, when they allow themselves to face their fears and to experience the things that are uncomfortable, they find true freedom inside. This enables them to be present and authentically happy.

Enneagram – Type 8

Type 8 is confident, commanding, and decisive. They know what they like and what they do not like. They can decide in seconds whether they like someone or not. They strive to be powerful and strong, and they get angry when their efforts to be strong are threatened. They do not mind if others find them intimidating. They resist weakness in themselves and others because to them this equals vulnerability, which is not acceptable. They do not mind following the rules if they agree with their instincts but happy to break them otherwise. When they decide on the way things are supposed to be, they will challenge anyone who takes on their will and authority. They enjoy winning and they are natural strategists. They are extremely resourceful and know how to get things done. They can be very impatient. They are very direct and sometimes they are shocked at how people are hurt by their directness. They do not actually mean to be hurtful, but they value honesty and they respect people who are direct. At their lowest, their response to betrayal is to take revenge. It is only as they evolve within their type that revenge would not be enacted but they will still cut someone out of their life if they betrayed them. At their stress point, they go to the worst of type 5 and need to be alone to decompress because their words can cut deep. At their best, they access the most desirable characteristics of type 2. They learn compassion and open their heart. Then they step into real power because they embrace vulnerability, realizing that makes them stronger. They become a benevolent generous leader with a big heart.

Enneagram – Type 9

Type 9 is easygoing on the surface, but they are an angry type. In fact, in some ways, they are asleep to their anger, and they

118

have an instinctive resistance to it. They do not let their anger surface because they are trying to be peaceful. Before they experience growth, they prefer to be hidden. They look for ways to numb themselves, to numb their feelings. They use routine to just tune out. They like the shell of okayness and peace. People describe them as quite chilled because they always seem okay. They will do anything to keep the peace, even if it means compromising themselves. They are not aware that they are doing that until they become more awake. It is only then that they experience real peace. In general, they are patient and non-judgmental. They can be very indecisive, and if you push them to make a decision, they can dig their heels in and procrastinate. They tend to ignore problems if they threaten to disturb their harmony and peace. They can be unaware of what they really need or want. When not evolved, this type tends to take on some of the worst characteristics of type 6, which means they procrastinate, overthink everything, and can be quite anxious. As they grow, they access the best characteristics of type 3. They come out of hiding, become action-orientated, realize what is important to them, and assert themselves in life. They find an honest relationship with anger, and they become a real embodiment of peace.

Are These Traits Something We Are Born with?

Before we move on from this topic, I want to say that I do not actually think that the Enneagram types are something we are born with. You may hear some people say that. I disagree. It is true that we can see those traits in young children, but in my opinion, what we are seeing are adaptations. After all, we develop adaptations from the moment we are born, and the first few years of life are key in shaping those adaptations.

We are not born perfectionists (type 1), people-pleasers (type 2), etc.

That said, I do think that we are born with different levels of resilience. In other words, we are born with different neurological susceptibilities that then dictate how we internally respond to external situations and what adaptations we develop as a result. These neurological susceptibilities or different levels of neurological resilience are influenced by many factors, including the mother's emotional state during pregnancy, the circumstances of birth, intergenerational trauma, etc. A neurologically weaker child will be more likely to interpret external stimuli as threats, which will then cause that child to develop the necessary adaptions to survive. A more resilient child may not have the need to develop that same adaptation because they do not have an internal stress response to that same external stimulus.

However, there is something else going on as well, I believe, with regards what personality type we end up with. It is our genetic imprint. To explain what I mean, I have to briefly mention a personality profiling method called Warriors, Settlers, and Nomads based on evolutionary psychology, developed by Terence Watts. I will describe it here very briefly to demonstrate the point I am making. Many thousands of years ago, human race was believed to have been split into two main genetic streams, hunters and gatherers, or Warriors and Nomads. When the first settlements started to appear, the third genetic stream evolved - Settlers.

These streams of genetic information survived through time, and we can definitely see these traits in every one of us. I believe these are traits we were actually born with. Or, to put it another way, there are three primary tendencies, which are our natural ways of being, inherited from our ancestors: Warrior (a natural leader, also methodical, organized, determined), Nomad (charismatic, outgoing, enthusiastic, uninhibited, a born entertainer), Settler (instinctive, caring, tolerant, flexible, passionate).

If you take two people with the same level of trauma, one may reinvent themselves and the other may go off the rails. Why? There is something innate in them that makes them choose one path or another. Those are the basic traits I just talked about. When I was born, my resilience was poor because my nervous system was in pieces, which made be susceptible to physical illness and subsequent emotional trauma. As a result, I developed some unhealthy adaptations that could have killed me, yet I survived. I bounced back. I remember the time when my inner Warrior woke up. I knew there was more to life than misery. Something deep inside wanted to fight for happiness, health, and emotional freedom. I went towards self-development and I rebalanced my mind and my nervous system. If my neurological state and adaptations I had developed were the only factors at play, I should have technically ended up on the street doing drugs. Some people would have in similar circumstances. But I did not. That is why I believe there is something else going on. I believe that we are born with those basic traits and predispositions, and we also develop those different adaptations in childhood, such as overachieving, overthinking, people-pleasing, withdrawal, perfectionism, and so on, in order to survive.

Now I recommend that you read through the Enneagram types again, thinking about the people closest to you, and see if you can figure out what types they are. This knowledge is very helpful when it comes to navigating relationships. Once you know your own type and your partner's or child's type, you can start adjusting your behavior and language if you want to avoid triggering them. The same applies to your work relationships. Recognizing somebody's type may mean you can get more out of that relationship.

Self-discovery with Transactional Analysis

Transactional Analysis (TA) is part of my method because I consider it extremely beneficial for getting to know what goes on in your psyche. There are many versions and levels of TA but we are going to keep it simple here, so you can start using it right away. However, before we explore TA, we need to make sure that we are on the same page with regards the ego.

The Concept of Ego

Many people understand many different things by *ego*, which makes the concept of ego confusing. The English word *ego* is the Latin word for *I*. Use of *ego* crept into psychology mostly through the work of Freud. In Freud's theory, the ego is the part of the personality that is positioned between the animalistic desires of the *id* and the moral and social standards of the *superego*. So Freud was referring to that conscious, decision-making part of you that you regard as *I*, e.g., *I dislike bananas* or *I decided to go on holiday*. In fact, when ego comes into play, you will often hear *I*, *me*, *mine*, *myself* being used.

Consider egoism, which means to act in one's self-interest. Someone who is behaving egoistically is simply pursuing his or her own goals. We all do that by the way at some level. Humans are inherently egocentric. Meaning, we can never break free from either our physical perspective (I can perceive the world only from my physical location in space), or our personal perspective that is influenced by our experiences, goals, beliefs, identities, preferences, and biases. Different people can to a lesser or greater degree step outside their own perspective to see things from other people's points of view. However, we are all stuck in a sense in our own egocentric viewpoint because there is no way we are able to process information, other than from our personal frame of reference. Clearly, just because you are honoring your needs and wants, does not mean you do not care about others. You can do both and be balanced about it. The problems arise when you are extreme about either everything being always about you, or always putting others first and completely ignoring your own needs.

What is interesting is that ego is often viewed in a negative way. But our ego is not really who we are. It is just a mask we put on for the world, and it is connected to the different roles we play. It is characterized by labels. The driver of the ego is fear and wanting to control. Whereas *your true self,* your higher self, is the field of infinite possibilities and creativity. The ego causes you to make choices based on how you are perceived by others or yourself. Any limiting beliefs will feed your ego. When you ask: *who am I?*, you might answer: *I am a mother, daughter, sister, animal lover, vegetarian, accountant.* These labels change all the time. Your true self, your spirit, or your energetic essence (this is NOTHING to do with religion) is not subject to such changes.

There are moments when you feel secure, accepted, peaceful and certain. At those moments, you are tapping into your true potential and the essence of you. At other moments, when you experience fear, insecurity, uncertainty, doubt, you are at the mercy of your ego-self. These two different realities produced by the same mind but the issue is that when you are in the ego-dominant state, you have difficulties even remembering who you actually are, and that you are capable of accessing your true potential and operating in a very different way. There will be times when you are doing this work and your mind comes up with doubts and excuses. *Am I doing it correctly? Am I on the right path? I don't have enough time to do this today.* Just acknowledge this is your ego showing up and carry on.

Practicing to gain some objectivity with regards to what is actually happening to you at any given moment makes it easier not to fall into those ego traps, where everything is frightening, unsafe and overwhelming. Because your ego is influenced by what goes on in the external world, it can get easily derailed, confused, agitated and disturbed. Your true self is stable, self-reliant, loving, creative, knowing, accepting, and peaceful. The reality is that whether you are in crisis, or need to solve a problem, it will serve you best to utilize the qualities of your true self. Easier said than done, right? If you currently feel like you have little or no access to this way of being and you are dominated by fear, insecurities, uncertainty, impulsiveness, survival instincts, and other qualities associated with your ego-self, just know that with this work you will be peeling off those layers and tapping into the essence of who you really are.

You may have heard people who are on a spiritual path saying that you need to destroy or erase the ego. However, for as long as you have a physical body, you will have an ego, just as much as you will have a mind and intellect. Rather than focusing on eliminating the ego, your aim should be to balance it so it acts in harmony with all your other layers of life. If we were born without ego, we simply would not survive and even if we would, we would be complete and utter doormats. Our ego serves a purpose. It shows up around the age of two. That is when we discover the word *mine*. Then, as we grow, the ego helps us stay away from danger and ensure our survival. It also supports us in our education, career, relationships, and dealing with life in general, as it loves to organize things. But, as we said, the dark side of the ego manifests as fear, arrogance, pride, vanity, judgements, prejudices, control, victimhood, the lust for power, fanaticism, or an obsession with materialism.

By the way, you may have heard the expression that someone has a "big ego." What this really means is high levels of insecurity and fear. People who stomp their feet with their chests puffed out in reality feel like a cornered wild animal fighting for their lives. The bottom line is that we can transcend the ego through building our self-awareness. We can also teach our ego humility through service to others and compassion. If we accept and love our ego, it will expand and cease to feel threatened. When we are more aware of our thoughts, feelings, behaviors, and language, choices we make and how our choices affect others, we begin to move beyond the ego and connect with who we truly are. We then start to live our lives more consciously, rather than being constantly hijacked by our ego.

Transactional Analysis in Practice

As I said, one of the tools that can help us become more aware of ourselves and others is TA, so let us explore it in more detail. TA was developed by Eric Berne following his training in psychoanalysis. Berne built upon Sigmund Freud's model of the *id*, *ego* and *super-ego*, and adapted post-Freudian Paul Federn's concepts of ego states. He supplemented Freud's ideas with observable behavior. TA is a psychoanalytic theory and method of therapy in which social interactions are analyzed to determine the ego state of the person as a basis for understanding and modifying behavior. Ego states refer to frames of mind we are in (encompassing thoughts, feelings and behavior) at a given time. Whilst each of us probably has thousands of ego states that change constantly, according to TA theory they all fit into one of three categories: Parent, Child and Adult.

TA explains that an individual's final emotional state is the result of inner dialogue between different parts of the psyche. This dialogue can of course be improved, therefore improving the emotional state of the person. TA also teaches us about the content of people's interactions with each other. Changing these interactions helps us solve emotional problems and/or conflicts. So basically, we can use this modality to get to know ourselves and improve how we manage what goes on inside our psyche, and we can also learn how to better navigate relationships. Let us now look in more detail at the three different ego states: Parent, Child and Adult.

Parent Ego State

This is a collection of subconscious recordings (programs) of external events perceived by us in our early years (in the first 5 years of our life). This is the time of our lives before we become socially engaged and aware, so the majority of those programs are provided by the example of our caregivers. Everything the child sees the caregivers do or hear them say is recorded in the Parent. There is a lot of "how to" data recorded here (survival skills). That data is taken in unquestioned and recorded without editing. The child's dependency, the inability to construct meaning with words, and to rationalize what is going on around them, makes it impossible for the child to modify or correct the information. Recorded in the Parent are all the rules and laws ("truths") that the caregivers live by. These can be positive (e.g., *touching a hot stove results in pain*) or negative (e.g., *emotions must not be expressed*). Those programs, or "truths", get replayed for the rest of the person's life unless they are recognized as unhelpful and changed.

Child Ego State

Whilst external events are being recorded as the body of data called the Parent, there is another recording being made simultaneously called the Child. This is the recording of internal responses of the child to what they see or hear. Since the child has no vocabulary during these most critical early experiences, most of their reactions are feelings. During this time of helplessness, when the child is small, inept, dependent, clumsy, and has no words to construct meaning, there are many demands on the child. On the one hand, the child has genetically coded urges to explore, to crush, to bang, to experience the surroundings. On the other hand, there is the constant demand from the environment (caregivers) that the child gives up on those urges in exchange for parental approval. The predominant by-product of this conflict is negative feelings experienced by the child. This in turn leads to the conclusion: *I'm not OK*. This happens to pretty much every child, even children of well-meaning and loving parents.

Adult Ego State

At about 10 months of age, the child learns to manipulate objects and begins to move more freely. They are also able to do things that grow from the child's own awareness. This self-actualization is the beginning of the Adult ego state. Adult data accumulates as a result of the child's ability to find out for themselves what is different about life from the *taught concept* of life stored in the Parent ego state and the *felt concept* of life recorded in the Child. The Adult is a new concept of life based on ongoing data gathering and data processing. During the early years, the Adult is fragile and can be easily suppressed by commands from the Parent ego state and fear coming from the Child ego state. Despite these interferences, the Adult continues to develop and progress. The Adult is essentially a data-processing center, which makes logical and rational decisions after computing the information from three sources: the Parent, the Child, and the data which the Adult has been gathering.

It is important to know that in TA we recognize two different aspects of both the Parent and the Child.

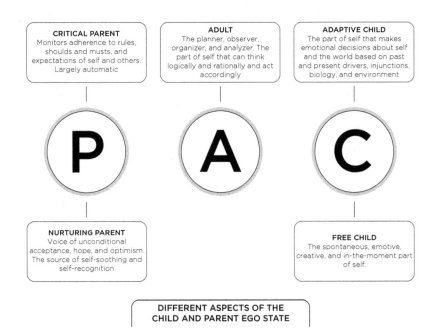

CRITICAL PARENT
Monitors adherence to rules, shoulds and musts, and expectations of self and others. Largely automatic

ADULT
The planner, observer, organizer, and analyzer. The part of self that can think logically and rationally and act accordingly

ADAPTIVE CHILD
The part of self that makes emotional decisions about self and the world based on past and present drivers, injunctions, biology, and environment

P   **A**   **C**

NURTURING PARENT
Voice of unconditional acceptance, hope, and optimism. The source of self-soothing and self-recognition

FREE CHILD
The spontaneous, emotive, creative, and in-the-moment part of self.

DIFFERENT ASPECTS OF THE CHILD AND PARENT EGO STATE

The Adaptive Child is the wounded part of the psyche that makes emotional decisions about self and the world based on unresolved trauma and limiting beliefs. This is the part that we need to heal. The other aspect of the Child is the Free Child, the creative, joyful, spontaneous part of our psyche that helps us be present. Likewise, we differentiate between the Critical Parent, the part of the psyche dominated by rules, *shoulds* and *musts*, and the Nurturing Parent, which is all about unconditional acceptance and self-love.

The Egogram Exercise

This exercise will help you assess which ego state(s) are currently dominant in your psyche and which may need to be strengthened. Below are some adjectives associated with each of the ego states. I would like you to assign numbers: 0, 1, 2, 3, or 4 to each adjective (0 = not at all accurate, 4 = extremely accurate). When you are scoring these adjectives think how you are being towards yourself in a stressed state. How are you treating yourself? Two important points before you start:

1. Make sure you are honest with yourself and assess where you are currently, not where you would like to be, or how you think others may see you. This is about being brutally honest with yourself.

2. A common mistake when doing this exercise is to start relating this to other people. So just to clarify, **this is nothing to do with other people**. This is about what goes on inside your own psyche, i.e. this is about how YOU feel about YOU.

Critical Parent	Nurturing Parent	Adult	Free Child	Adapted Child
Autocratic	Affectionate	Alert	Adventurous	Anxious
Bossy	Considerate	Capable	Affectionate	Apathetic
Demanding	Forgiving	Clear-thinking	Artistic	Argumentative
Dominant	Generous	Efficient	Energetic	Arrogant
Fault-seeking	Gentle	Fair-minded	Enthusiastic	Awkward
Forceful	Helpful	Logical	Excitable	Complaining
Intolerant	Kind	Methodical	Humorous	Confused
Nagging	Praising	Organised	Imaginative	Defensive
Opinionated	Sympathetic	Precise	Natural	Dependent
Prejudiced	Tolerant	Rational	Pleasure-seeking	Inhibited
Rigid	Understanding	Realistic	Spontaneous	Moody
Severe	Unselfish	Reasonable	Uninhibited	Easily stressed
Stern	Warm	Unemotional	Care-free	Chaotic

Egogram Exercise

I have to be a bit blunt again at this point. This is because I want to make sure you are not cheating yourself out of an awakening here. If you are reading this book because you feel something at the psycho-energetic level is blocking your healing and yet you go through this exercise and score the highest for the Nurturing Parent and/or the Free Child, something is not right. You either have a very low level of self-awareness, you are completely disconnected from reality, and/or you are lying to yourself. Why do I say this? Because if your Parent ego state were amazingly nurturing and your Child ego state were wonderfully free, you would not be here reading this book trying to get answers for what you are experiencing. This book would not even be on your radar because you would be a happy, healthy, resilient, super-aligned individual.

Most people reading this book are doing so because they know they have work to do. If you identify with that, your Parent will be at this time predominantly critical and your

Child will be predominantly wounded. Clearly, you want to aim for your Parent to be nurturing and your Child to be free. That is absolutely the aim of this work. However, this is unlikely to be the case when you are just starting to address your psycho-energetic health. If you are already partly there, that is wonderful. If you are currently dominated by your Critical Parent and your Adaptive Child, that is fine too. That is exactly why you are here doing this work.

The reason some people may be inclined to give high scores to the adjectives that sound better is because when they give high scores to those adjectives that do not sound so good, they are looking at their own shadow. They may get resistance to giving a high score to what they do not want to be or do not want to be associated with. But please be honest about how you are treating yourself at this point in time. Look at it, own it, have no attachment to it, but accept that you have some work to do. That is absolutely fine. Like I said, your scores for the Nurturing Parent and the Free Child may be low right now, or may even be zero. That is OK. This just shows you where you need to focus to improve.

Now that you have scored the adjectives, plot your results on a graph. This is called an Egogram. You can see an example of it below. Construct yours based on your own scores. What you need to know about this Egogram is that, when one state increases in intensity, the others will decrease to compensate. There is a shift in psychic energies but the total energy in the system remains the same. As we progress through the method and you will work on various aspects of your psycho-energetic healing, these scores will start to change. To begin with, on a cognitive level, the way to achieve a positive shift is to think which part you want to be more prominent and act accordingly.

The adjectives associated with that part will prompt you as to different behaviors you can practice. When you do that, the energy will automatically shift out of the other states that you want to be less dominant into the states that you want to be more dominant.

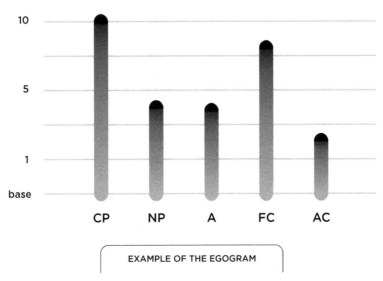

EXAMPLE OF THE EGOGRAM

So just to summarize, when you are being critical of yourself or others, when you are hard on yourself, beating yourself up, telling yourself (or others) off, or regurgitating what your parents used to say all the time, your Critical Parent is being dominant in those moments. When you are being emotional, scared, hurt, feeling stupid, unworthy, etc., when you are "having a tantrum", that is your Adaptive (Wounded) Child talking. When you are seeing things for what they are, being matter-of-fact, objective, logical and rational, you are being in your Adult ego state.

Depending on the circumstances, you always switch back and forth between your ego states. Unless you have done much self-development work, you will frequently have your ego states fighting inside your head creating inner conflict, which is one of the biggest sources of emotional toxicity. Those internal conflicts are because of the different parts of the psyche not agreeing. Often this will be between your Child and your Adult, or your Parent and your Adult. Your Parent and your Child operate at the subconscious level, whereas your Adult is more of a conscious mind concept. So when you have those moments of battle between your conscious and subconscious, it is a conversation between your Child and Adult, or your Parent and Adult ego states. However, those disagreements can also happen between the Parent and the Child as well. Often those exchanges go back and forth.

Below are a few examples of exchanges that may take place inside somebody's mind. Hopefully, this further illustrates how we switch between those different states constantly. Mostly, people do this without any awareness but now that you understand the different parts and their roles, you can choose to engage a different part of your psyche when you get caught up having an argument with yourself.

Adaptive Child (AC) - Adult (A)
AC: *I can't go to this party. They will not like me.*
A: *I am being silly. They don't even know me, so I can't assume they will not like me in advance. This doesn't make any sense.*

Critical Parent (CP) - Adult (A)
CP: *I can't believe I made such a stupid mistake!*
A: *Oh well. Everybody makes mistakes. It is a fact of life. I can learn from it and get it right next time. No big deal.*

Critical Parent (CP) - Adaptive child (AC)
CP: *I have to be more assertive when talking to people.*

AC: But I don't think I've got it in me. Plus, what if they won't like me anymore?

Critical Parent (CP) - Free child (FC)
CP: *I really should do this.*
FC: *But I don't want to right now. I'd rather do something fun instead.*

Adaptive Child (AC) - Nurturing parent (NP)
AC: *I am really angry at Anna for saying those things.*
NP: *I am sure she did not mean to hurt my feelings but it is OK for me to feel angry.*

So what we essentially seek to do with this modality is to reframe our subconscious thought processes. We seek to discover an understanding of which part of the psyche is running a given program and why. Then, we can rechannel the needs and requirements of that part into a more constructive and useful behavior pattern. This is obviously not an ultimate panaceum but it is one of the tools we can utilize to reprogram the subconscious.

Action Points:

In addition to continuing with the tasks from Chapter 1:

1. Write down in a journal your scores for the two parts of the Emotional Toxicity Questionnaire (the first part is where you are going to see the shifts as you make progress), as well as your reflections on what you have discovered about your attachment style and your Enneagram type. Even if you are still unsure at this point, just write down what you think those are and why you think that.

2. Write down your reflections on what you think your secondary gain is. If you are unsure at this point, take a guess what it might be.

3. Identify a few behaviors based on the list of adjectives in the Egogram exercise that will help you increase the activity of your Nurturing Parent and your Free Child and start implementing those.

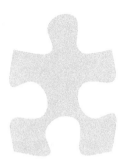

Resilience & the Nervous System Balance

Different Types of Resilience & Resilience Traits

Kate had suffered from digestive problems and immune issues for almost ten years before she approached me to work with her. She had every single digestive symptom you can think of, which made her miserable and interfered greatly with her personal, professional, and social life. She had three autoimmune diagnoses and multiple food sensitivities. She had been treated for SIBO, IBS, and her autoimmune issues by multiple practitioners over the years, but all the efforts and sacrifice resulted in only partial success. She had even gone to the famous Cleveland Clinic, which again did not amount to much. Even though Kate had periods of time when she would do a little better, ultimately, she would always end up circling back to more or less where she had started from. In addition to spending tens of thousands of dollars on practitioners and specialists, she also spent a crazy amount of money on supplements. She had become obsessed with having to try any new supplement she would read or hear about in the hope that would be her breakthrough. However, her body just would not tolerate most of those products. This was despite them being of superb quality and recommended by some of the top autoimmune experts in the online health space. Kate had gone through periods of depression but luckily, she was not going to give up. Something was telling her that there was a solution and that she simply had not found it yet. She was determined to get better, and she was hungry for knowledge.

One day, she was attending an online summit at which I happened to be speaking. I talked about the nervous system balance and how it was not possible to fully heal immune and digestive issues without addressing nervous system dysregulation. Kate knew immediately that this was her missing link. She contacted me to help her, and we arranged our first session. Similarly to many of my clients, Kate had a history of complex trauma that caused her to be very emotionally toxic, which, over time, resulted in the breakdown of her physical body. Among other things, she suffered satanic ritualistic abuse as a child. Safety was not much of a feature of Kate's childhood. She had a narcissistic father, and her mother was too scared to protect her. This resulted in chronic anxiety with periods of depression, self-loathing, lack of self-confidence, and a string of toxic relationships in her adult life. No wonder her nervous as well as her immune system were completely dysregulated. Her partner had little understanding for what she was going through physically and mentally, and he was highly demanding and critical. As Kate already had a great deal of self-loathing, any criticism from her partner and his endless demands of her to do everything better, faster, or more efficiently would trigger her to self-destruct. In response, she would binge on junk food to numb herself, knowing this was going to cause her body to flare up, and then she would hate herself for causing those setbacks.

When we started to work together, Kate was desperate to break that vicious cycle. Within six to eight sessions of addressing her emotional toxicity and the resulting nervous system imbalance, Kate was noticing changes not only at the emotional level but she also started observing significant improvements in her physical symptoms. It is important to note that Kate was very committed to doing her daily homework, which my clients are always prescribed, and that it was putting all the work in between our sessions that enabled her to get very profound results as quickly as she did.

One of the first things she noticed was improved gut function and decreased inflammation. At that point, she decided to try one of the supplements she had not been previously able to tolerate that she still had in her cupboard. She did not have an adverse gut reaction to it, so she was able to introduce it and finally started to benefit from it. Kate was very encouraged by that and decided to put her gut to another test. She was invited a party and she tried a few food items from the buffet that would normally make her sick for a number of days. I would not usually advise such experiments, but she was adamant that she needed to know how she was going to respond. She was ecstatic when the normal response of nausea, bloating, and extreme fatigue the following day did not materialize. We continued to work together for a few more weeks, by which time she had all the tools and confidence she needed to carry on the work on her own. She emailed me at some point to say that she had decided to leave her relationship. She said she had come to the conclusion that she deserved much better than being in a relationship with a narcissist.

Now that she really knew her worth, Kate was not going to reproduce that same old pattern again. This was a major breakthrough for Kate and in some way a culmination of all the self-development work. Her emotional toxicity score decreased dramatically, which meant her nervous system and her physical body were able to start to rebalance and function correctly. Over the years, I have worked with many clients like Kate. Kate's and others' experiences demonstrate what a destructive effect a dysregulated nervous system that originates from early exposure to stress and early trauma can have, and also that it is possible to turn it around.

What Does It Mean to Be Resilient?

When we talk about resilience, we are talking about bouncing back quickly from any life difficulties so that the adversity does not define us in any way, or ruin our mental and physical health. Being resilient is absolutely essential if you want optimal health long-term because life will always happen and there will always be unpleasant surprises and trauma as we move through it. Without resilience we are very fragile mentally and physically. The reality is that we cannot control the external. However, we can 100 percent control our response to whatever is going on in the external. We can make sure that we become so robust that we can always respond to any circumstances in a way that is not destructive to our health and well-being.

Those who master resilience are able to face emergencies and accept what comes at them with flexibility rather than rigidity. This behavioral flexibility is a key feature of resilience. The old adage applies here: *Resilient people are like bamboo in a hurricane—they bend rather than break.* Or, even if they feel like they are broken for a period time, they know it is temporary and know that they will not be broken forever. We have already mentioned nervous system balance is critical to health and healing, meaning it affects how physically resilient you are. In this chapter, we will focus on resilience from a neurological perspective. I share strategies that can help you improve nervous system balance via addressing vagal tone.

In addition, I talk about emotional resilience, which, of course, is also key to our physical well-being. Emotional and neurological resilience are interconnected. It is really just a different way of viewing resilience. When we are emotionally resilient, we have control over our emotions. There will be a whole chapter dedicated to emotional mastery in this book, but for now, I would like to emphasize that you cannot have emotional resilience without neurological resilience. Meaning, if you are wired to constantly activate the fight, flight, or freeze response, you will have a really hard time managing your emotions. You can, however, use emotional work to correct that nervous system imbalance.

On the other hand, when you have healthy emotional responses, you will be doing well on a neurological level. You then just need to consider all the other stressors that are putting a strain on your nervous system, such as chemical toxins, biological agents (bacteria, viruses, parasites, mold, etc.), certain foods (depending on what your immune system perceives as a threat), EMFs, and physical (mechanical) stressors, such as spinal subluxations. Those additional factors are not the focus of this book, but I do want you to be aware of them, as they do contribute to the nervous system imbalance, which decreases neurological resilience.

Our energy field also contributes to our resilience, so we will be looking at that later in the book. There is also spirituality. When you believe that you are part of something greater than yourself, and that there is more to our existence than just this physical reality, you can access a higher level of resilience that non-spiritual people do not have access to.

Traits of Resilient People

As we are looking at the key traits of resilient people, I will be asking you some questions to help you identify where you may need to put more emphasis in order to increase your resilience.

Behavioral Flexibility

This is incredibly important if you want to be resilient, so ask yourself: when you have a plan of where you are going and you are faced with a difficulty, do you resist the obstacle, or do you say: *OK, that's fine. I will go down a different path instead?* Do you break down, scream and shout, and feel victimized, or do you pick yourself up, dust yourself off, and decide what to do next, and where to go next, with ease and grace? Even if you initially feel knocked out by what happened, how long does it take you to pick yourself up and keep going?

Seeing Difficulties as Temporary

Resilient people do not identify with their difficulties. They understand that there is a separation between who they are at their core and the cause of their temporary suffering. Even though stress or trauma might play a part in their story, it does not interfere with their identity. So ask yourself: How strongly do you identify with your traumas and difficult circumstances in life? When something goes "wrong" in your life, does it feel

141

like it is here to stay? Like it is insurmountable? Like you will never be able to recover from it? I know this depends how serious something is in your perception, but think about those really bad moments. Do you feel engulfed by those difficulties? Does it ever feel permanent? It is normal to feel down initially when something bad happens, but I am referring to a feeling of permanence, as though things are never going to get better.

Self-Awareness

Resilient people are self-aware, which is why there is so much emphasis on it in my method. Being blissfully unaware can get us through a bad day, but it is not a good long-term strategy. Being self-aware means we are in touch with our psychological, emotional, and physiological needs. It means knowing what we need, what we do not need, and when it is time to ask for help. Self-awareness is about being good at listening to the subtle cues your body and mind are sending. So how good are you at identifying your emotional and physical needs right now?

Asking for Help

Resilient people understand that being resilient is not about always doing everything themselves and having to conquer the world on their own. Stubbornness without any flexibility or self-awareness does not do us any good. We have to be able to ask for help sometimes and be OK with that. Not wanting to ask for help does not necessarily make you strong. If by not asking for help you are cutting your nose to spite your face, then it actually makes you weak. So how good are you at asking for help when you are faced with difficulties and you feel like you are struggling to cope?

Practicing Acceptance & Embracing Change

Acceptance is not about giving up and letting the stress take over. It is about allowing yourself to experience the full range of emotions and trusting that you will bounce back. Again, it is resistance that makes the pain and suffering worse. Resilient people know how to be in flow. They understand that stress and discomfort is part of our experience here in this physical realm, and they understand that ignoring, repressing, or denying emotions makes everything worse. Unfortunately, people have a tendency to hold on to the familiar, even when it is terrible and traumatic. The human nervous system likes familiarity. When people are not very resilient, they want to hold on to the familiar at all costs.

Resilience means accepting what is and embracing change. It also means being confident going in a new direction—one that you create. For humans, letting go is clearly a process, and it is not necessarily human nature to want to let things go, but the alternative does not serve us well. It is very stressful. I would like to point out that this is not about giving yourself a hard time that you have not yet accepted your circumstances. Everybody will grieve after the old and familiar at a different pace. But it is not until we accept our current reality that we can move on, and being resilient means getting there faster. So how quickly do you accept things for what they are when life happens? How quickly can you usually accept your circumstances and start moving on?

Perceptions & "Truths" Are Not Set in Stone

Because resilient people are flexible, they can expand their map of the world easily, so they don't struggle to accept new truths and reject old ones. A truth is only your truth until it stops being your truth. So the question is: how easy is it for you to consider other points of view outside of what you are currently believing? Think to when you have conversations with people and they bring up a point you have not considered before. Do you dismiss that as invalid because it is not your truth, or do you consider it carefully?

Being Silent

Resilient people are able and willing to be silent. Many people are addicted to distractions: TV, shopping, family, work, over-eating, drugs, taking risks, gossip, etc. They tell themselves they need those behaviors, but it is just an excuse not go inside. When you become more resilient, you have no issue meditating or spending time on your own. So the question is: how good are you currently at being still and silent or spending time on your own? Do you need distractions?

Relinquishing Control

Resilient people do not need to control every last little aspect of their lives. Being resilient means trusting that you can fig-ure life out as it happens. The negative bias means humans have this tendency not only to register negative stimuli more readily but also to dwell on these events. That makes people pessimistic and fearful, wanting to be "prepared" when bad things happen. However, when you are resilient, you have more trust in your own ability to handle life, whatever it may bring you. This means you do not need that safety blanket of pes-simism and fear, which in itself is a stressor and emotionally toxic. So do you go with the flow, trusting you will be able to handle what comes your way? Or do you feel like you need to control your life as much as possible? Do you have an urge to plan everything in great detail because you feel that helps you prepare for what may be coming?

Not Sweating the Small Stuff

Resilient people do not go into the stress response over the tiniest things. That is because they have trained their nervous systems to make sure they do not get hijacked by their fight-or-flight response. They do understand that it is OK to feel fear, anger, or whatever else, but they do not stay in that response. They have learned to move through and out of it easily. How easy is it for you to come back to feeling relaxed after something stressful happens? How long does it usually take you to drop into that parasympathetic rest-digest-detoxify-heal response?

Taking Responsibility

Resilient people are not stuck in victimhood. They take owner-ship. When you allow yourself to be a victim, when you choose victimhood, you are perpetuating your stress, and therefore you are perpetuating your physical issues. Are you feeling victim-ized right now by what you are experiencing, for example, your health or work situation, your relationship, etc.? Do you blame anybody for anything that is not right in your life? Blaming and pointing a finger at other people means you are suffering from what I describe as *chronic victimitis*. If you tend to blame others for what is not right in your life, I recommend that for now you just set an intention to step out of victimhood.

Maintenance & Self-Care

Resilience should not be taken for granted. You have to put energy into building resilience in the first place and then you need to maintain what you have built. It is important to understand the value of self-care and have your go-to strategies that recharge your batteries. So how good are you at self-care right now?

Ways to Affirm Resilience

Hopefully, you now have a better understanding of which of those areas you may have work to do in order to make yourself more resilient. In summary, resilience ultimately means believing:

I am OK.
I will be OK.
I can get through this.
It is an experience.
I am here to experience.
This too shall pass.

The Vagus Nerve & Its Role in Health & Healing

I have mentioned the importance of our nervous system being balanced on a number of occasions already. Let us know have a closer look at the different branches of the nervous system and some simple ways in which you can start to optimize your nervous system function. Just as a reminder, our nervous system consists of two main parts: the central nervous system (CNS) and the peripheral nervous system (PNS). The central nervous system consists of the brain and spinal cord. The peripheral nervous system is divided into the somatic nervous system and the autonomic nervous system.

The somatic nervous system controls all voluntary muscular systems within the body, whereas all the functions we do not have to consciously control are carried out by the autonomic nervous system. Finally, the autonomic nervous system is divided into the sympathetic and parasympathetic nervous system. You can think of these two branches as the gas and brake pedals in your car, respectively.

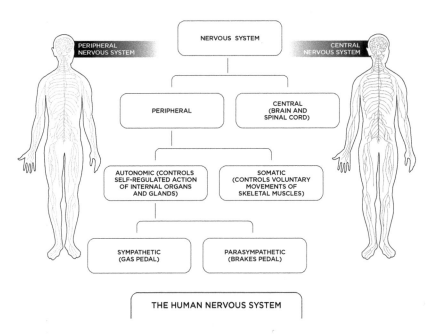

For now, we are going to focus on the autonomic nervous system and how we can balance its different branches to achieve better neurological stability. The sympathetic nervous system is associated with the fight-or-flight response, whereas the parasympathetic control of the body is carried out by the vagus nerve. The name *vagus* in Latin means *wandering*. The vagus nerve originates in the brainstem. It is the tenth cranial nerve, the longest nerve of the autonomic nervous system and one of the most important nerves in the body. The vagus nerve is responsible for the parasympathetic control of the majority of our internal organs, including our heart, lungs, stomach, pancreas, gallbladder, liver, small intestine, large intestine (the first two-thirds of it), thymus, and spleen. So this means the vagus nerve connects the brain with almost every organ in your body!

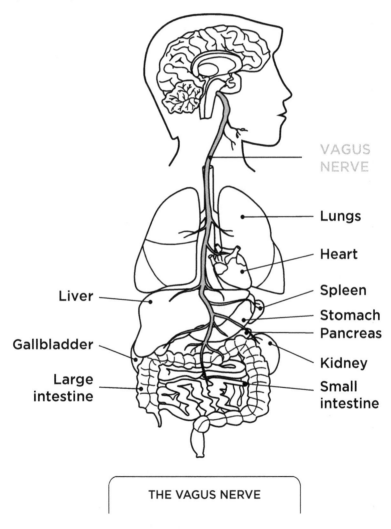

THE VAGUS NERVE

The vagus nerves are normally referred to in the singular, but there are actually two of them. The dorsal vagal complex (DVC) is the more primitive, unmyelinated branch of the vagus nerve, and its activation is what is known as the freeze response. The ventral vagal complex (VVC) is the newer myelinated branch of the vagus nerve that developed in mammals, and it is known as our social engagement system. Dr. Stephen Porges, the developer of the Polyvagal Theory, describes a three-part hierarchical response to stress or danger: ventral vagus activation (relaxation and social engagement), sympathetic activation (fight or flight), and dorsal vagus activation (immobilization or freeze).

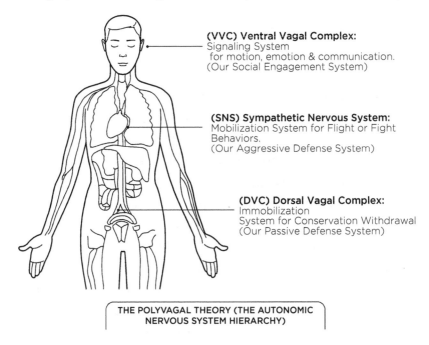

(VVC) Ventral Vagal Complex:
Signaling System
for motion, emotion & communication.
(Our Social Engagement System)

(SNS) Sympathetic Nervous System:
Mobilization System for Flight or Fight Behaviors.
(Our Aggressive Defense System)

(DVC) Dorsal Vagal Complex:
Immobilization
System for Conservation Withdrawal
(Our Passive Defense System)

THE POLYVAGAL THEORY (THE AUTONOMIC NERVOUS SYSTEM HIERARCHY)

During non-stressful situations, if we are emotionally healthy, our bodies stay in a social engagement state, or a happy, normal, relaxed state. This is our rest-and-digest response or, as I like to call it, our rest-digest-detoxify-heal response. In this state we are capable of connecting with others. On the other hand, the sympathetic nervous system is our immediate reaction to stress that affects nearly every organ in the body. The resulting fight-or-flight state is designed to keep us alive. In fight-or-flight, at some level, we believe we can still survive the threat we are facing in that moment. But when our sympathetic nervous system has kicked into overdrive and we are still unable to escape (flight) or defeat the threat in a fight, the dorsal branch of the vagus nerve takes control. This causes freezing or shutdown and is a form of self-preservation. Depending on the severity of the situation, this could be someone passing out under extreme stress, or somebody freezing on stage, unable to get their words out.

I have previously mentioned that we have evolved to live predominantly in a relaxed state, activate the fight, flight or freeze response when we face danger, and then re-activate the relaxation response after the danger has passed. So the problem is not accessing those survival states per sé because they are there for good reasons and they help us survive. The issues arise when we access those states too frequently or get stuck in them, which many people do due to unresolved traumas, chronic negative emotional states, limiting beliefs, poor self-worth, and day-to-day stress. Add to this all the other types of stressors, such as chemical toxins, EMFs, foods people are sensitive to, and so on, and we are dealing with chronic activation of those survival responses, in which no healing or regeneration takes place. As we already said:

WE CAN ONLY HEAL WHEN WE SPEND ENOUGH TIME IN THE RELAXATION RESPONSE.

FIGHT FLIGHT FREEZE

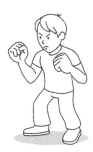 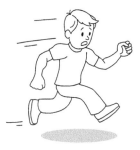 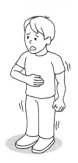

WHEN SURVIVAL IS PRIORITY HEALING IS A BACKSEAT ISSUE

SURVIVAL STATES AND HEALING

The more the nervous system is trained to activate the fight, flight, or freeze response, the better it becomes at activating those responses, and the more challenged it feels when it comes to the ventral vagus activation. This is what I am talking about when I talk about autonomic nervous system imbalance. As the vagus nerve activates less frequently, it loses its tone, which is why we describe poor vagus nerve function as low vagal tone. Because the vagus nerve innervates all of those different organs, low vagal tone has been linked to many different health issues, including:

- chronic inflammation (via cholinergic anti-inflammatory pathway)
- chronic fatigue (low vagal tone is associated with decreased mitochondrial function)
- increased sensitivity to foods, chemicals, EMFs, etc.

151

- decreased ability to fight infections
- decreases ability to neutralize and remove toxins
- hormonal imbalances
- digestive problems, such as: IBS, IBD, SIBO, SIFO, leaky gut, dysbiosis, decreased stomach acid and/or digestive enzymes, abdominal bloating or pain, bowel transit time less than 10 hours or more than 20 hours (often resulting in diarrhea or constipation)
- depression/anxiety
- Alzheimer's
- Parkinson's
- PTSD
- thyroid disorders
- heart disease, abnormal heart rate and/or blood pressure
- dysglycaemia as well as diabetes
- chronic pain
- migraines and cluster headaches
- ADHD
- autoimmune disease, such as rheumatoid arthritis, multiple sclerosis, lupus, etc.
- obesity
- cancer (low vagal tone means much poorer prognosis)
- asthma
- difficulty speaking or loss of voice
- a voice that is hoarse, wheezy, or monotone
- difficulty drinking liquids
- loss of the gag reflex
- brain fog and memory problems.

Different Factors That Contribute to Poor Vagus Function

I have already discussed why I believe that emotional toxicity, which is synonymous with chronic stress, is one of the key contributing factors to nervous system dysfunction. However, there also other factors that affect our nervous systems and contribute to low vagal tone.

Dysfunctional Breathing

If your pattern of breathing is dysfunctional, which is the case for many people, you will be constantly sending a message to your brain that there is something wrong. Many people's breathing is restricted to their upper chests, and they hold their breath for a portion of the breathing cycle. If that is how you breathe habitually, your sympathetic nervous system will be activating when it does not need to because we normally switch to shallow, erratic breathing when we are in stressful situations. This will, over time, lower your vagal tone. The same is true if you breathe through your mouth all the time, which again is very common. For most people with dysfunctional breathing patterns, this problem goes back to their birth or early trauma. The original loss of functionality is then reinforced over time. It is possible to learn how to breathe properly. If you have a tendency to breathe through your mouth, you can try taping your mouth at night to force yourself to breathe through your nose and prevent heightened brain activity during sleep.

Dysfunctional Digestion

The digestive sequence is under vagus nerve control. It is quite complex, and when even the smallest aspect of it is off, the whole sequence is disrupted. In addition, anything that negatively affects any organs that form part of the digestive process

153

will contribute to overall dysfunction. So eating toxic foods (and living a toxic lifestyle), eating too fast or in a stressed state, not chewing properly, etc., will all lead to a disrupted digestive sequence, organ insufficiency (e.g., liver, gall bladder, pancreas), gut inflammation, leaky gut, and dysbiosis. This, in turn, leads to reduced vagus function due to this back and forth communication that occurs between the gut and the brain.

Chronic Inflammation

As previously mentioned, chronic inflammation is one of the most obvious signs of poor vagus nerve function. There are obviously many causes of chronic inflammation but wherever it is coming from, the vagus nerve should be able to turn it off. The more chronic inflammation builds up and the more the vagus nerve struggles, the more ineffective it becomes at putting the brakes on inflammation. This can become a real vicious cycle.

Dysfunctional Heart Rate

People whose heart rate is always higher than it should be for any given situation (e.g., at rest), constantly shut down their vagus nerve, and when the vagus is not activated enough, it stops working properly. Some of the best techniques that can help you positively change that are slow deep breathing, meditation (provided you respond well to it), and physical exercise.

Dysfunctional Sleep & Circadian Rhythm

Vagus nerve activity is supposed to be higher during stages 3 and 4 of sleep, but that will not happen if your sleep and circadian rhythms are not optimized. As it happens, circadian rhythms influence many aspects of health, including hormonal balance, mitochondrial function, and cellular detox. Any circadian dysregulation will have a negative knock-on effect on the vagus nerve. Remember that even though circadian rhythms are endogenously generated, they can be modulated by external cues such as light, temperature, food timing, and physical activity timing. So, making sure that your sleep is restorative is more complex than just getting eight hours of sleep per night. It is essential to have a good sleep hygiene routine and address any underlying causes of sleep dysfunction, which often is emotional toxicity. Again, this tends to be a vicious cycle for many people.

Infections

Not many people realize that the vagus nerve can be infected. Dr. Michael VanElzakker proposes that certain biological agents can affect the vagus nerve and trigger an exaggerated immune response that produces symptom clusters that we see frequently in chronic illnesses. Those symptoms include fatigue, fever, pain, brain fog, and depression. The vagus nerve can get infected via the oral cavity (via the trigeminal nerve), through latent infections when immunity is lowered, or as a result of an acute infection. Some of those biological agents include different viruses with high affinity for nerves, such as Epstein Barr or herpes viruses, but also Borrelia spirochetes.

Toxicity

The vagus nerve can also be toxic. Toxins have a particularly high affinity for our nerves, and toxic metals are among the most toxic agents, which also take the longest to detoxify. We are bombarded by toxins. They are in our air, water, and food chain. In addition, conventional cleaning and personal care products (this includes toothpaste), cookware, plasticware, furniture, carpets, paints, and most fabrics and dyes are toxic. So yes, we do have a sophisticated detoxification system, BUT our body's system is not able to adapt to all the man-made chemicals that have been introduced into our environment in the last few decades, which is in the region of 50 million. In addition, our oral cavity can be a huge source of toxicity for the vagus nerve, again via the trigeminal nerve, so if you think that may be a contributing factor for you, please look into that more.

Vagus Nerve & Immunity

Because of the very close connection between our nervous system function and our immune function, if our autonomic nervous system balance is disrupted, our immune function will also be dysregulated. This is, of course, bad news when an infection comes along. In contrast, people with a stronger vagus response recover more quickly after illness, injury, emotional trauma, or stress. The immune system is our defence system. It comprises many biological structures and processes that protect us against disease. Most people know that. What most people do not know is that the process to keep the immune system in check is mediated through the vagus nerve. Only when the vagus nerve is functioning well is it able to activate the cholinergic anti-inflammatory pathway. This is the pathway that puts the brakes on inflammation once inflammation has served its purpose. Acute inflammation is an appropriate immune response, but chronic inflammation is not, and chronic inflammation is a feature of pretty much every chronic illness.

Research shows that inflammatory conditions, such as rheumatoid arthritis, fibromyalgia, depression, etc., are associated with decreased heart rate variability, which is a marker of reduced vagal tone. This is connected to high levels of pro-inflammatory cytokines and an increase in sympathetic nervous system activity and stress hormones, which contribute to systemic inflammation. This happens because the vagus nerve is not strong enough to shut the inflammation off.

In addition, as we already said, the vagus nerve innervates the immune organs, such as the spleen, the thymus, and the gut. Those organs require strong vagus activity to keep them active. Constantly activating the fight, flight, or freeze response shuts down the activity of these organs. Decreased activity of the spleen means poor filtration of white and red blood cells. An underactive spleen also stops being effective at detecting viruses, bacteria and other pathogens, which is one of the key jobs of this immune organ. As for the thymus, this immune organ is primarily involved in the production of T cells. The body uses T cells to destroy infected or cancerous cells. T cells also help other organs in the immune system grow properly. It is true that we lose thymus activity as we age (involution of the thymus), but people's chronically stressful and toxic lifestyles, leading to poor vagal tone, cause the thymus to deactivate earlier than it should. This again results in increased risk of viral and bacterial infections. It is also one of the root causes of autoimmunity.

Then, there is the gut. The vagus nerve is the main digestive nerve, and your digestive system depends on it for proper function. Pretty much every aspect of normal digestion—secretion of gastric juices, motility (movement of the foods and stool), and nutrient absorption—is dependent on proper vagus nerve function. Without the vagus nerve functioning properly, food and stool does not pass through the intestines normally and the digestive process is impaired. Digestion actually begins in the brain via the vagus nerve long before food is even ingested and mechanically broken down in the mouth. This nerve facilitates the brain speaking to the body to initiate digesting food and releasing bile and acids for digestion, as well as to trigger the Migrating Motor Complex (MMC). When that communication is in any way compromised, the body may not know when to digest food or when to move food and bacteria through the intestines. This can create the right environment for small intestinal bacterial overgrowth (SIBO) to develop.

You may have heard that 70 to 80 percent of our immune system is in the gut. But why is that? Because this is the easiest way for any pathogens to enter the body due to the direct link to the outside environment. So, therefore, the great majority of our immune cells are found in the lining of the gut. This is known as gut-associated lymphoid tissue (GALT). The gut microbiome helps regulate the inflammatory response and it also affects the brain. This is why you often hear that gut health is the basis of health and that gut dysfunction is the root cause of many chronic diseases. As you already know, I argue that this is only partially correct. And here is why I say that.

The way the gut communicates with the brain is via the vagus nerve, as this nerve is the main component of the gut-brain axis. The vagus nerve is the information super-highway, and without it the gut and microbiome impact are actually quite limited. This has been demonstrated in studies that involved administering specific bacterial strains Bifidobacterium longum and Lactobacillus rhamnosus. In those separate studies, they have clearly showed the vagus nerve involvement. In mice with a severed vagus nerve (vagotomized), the effect of the micro-organisms and the gut-brain communication was drastically reduced. In fact, it pretty much ceased.

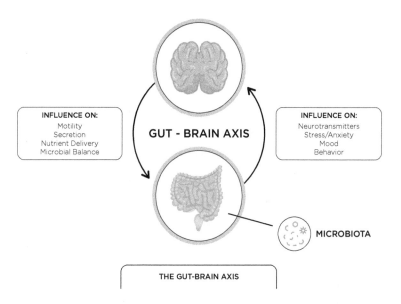

INFLUENCE ON:
Motility
Secretion
Nutrient Delivery
Microbial Balance

GUT - BRAIN AXIS

INFLUENCE ON:
Neurotransmitters
Stress/Anxiety
Mood
Behavior

MICROBIOTA

THE GUT-BRAIN AXIS

When immune cells first detect the presence of patho-
genic or toxic agents in the gut, the vagus nerve stimulates
the thymus and the spleen to increase their activity. At the
same time, the stress response and the sympathetic nerves
are activated, which causes the release of the neurotransmitter norepinephrine. This, in turn, causes the immune system
to be highly reactive to the threat. When the threat has been
dealt with, the reactivity is halted by the vagus nerve, which
is supposed to turn off that immune response since it is no
longer needed. A different neurotransmitter, acetylcholine, is
released to act on the gut and other parts of the body. This is
what keeps the immune reactivity in check, but this system
only works well when there is enough capacity to turn the
response off.

So it is about more than just the gut. We have seen this in
the research, and I can 100 percent confirm from my clinical
experience, that strengthening the vagus nerve improves gut

issues, as well as many other health problems. I know many other practitioners who can confirm that as well. In fact, when nervous system dysfunction is addressed at the root cause, this can often completely eliminate physical symptoms. Plus, this explains why many people have been working really hard to heal their gut for years, have tried every protocol and every supplement under the sun, and they are still not where they want to be. A dysregulated nervous system and poor vagal tone is a major link they are missing. Interestingly, when this is fixed, suddenly, these people feel like their diet and supplements are suddenly working. This is because they are finally able to break them down and assimilate them properly. So the bottom line is this:

YOU WILL STRUGGLE TO ACHIEVE OPTIMAL GUT FUNCTION WITHOUT A WELL-FUCTIONING VAGUS NERVE, REGARDLESS OF HOW CLEAN AND ORGANIC YOUR DIET IS OR HOW MANY SUPPLEMENTS YOU TAKE.

Treating the Untreatable with Vagus Nerve Stimulation

There are more and more research studies that clearly demonstrate what can be achieved with vagus nerve stimulation and restoring a healthy vagus nerve function. In 2012, Dr. Kevin Tracey, a professor of neurosurgery and molecular medicine, reported that electrically stimulating the vagus nerve of a patient with debilitating rheumatoid arthritis produced extraordinary results. The patient was in *clinical remission* within eight weeks of implanting an electrical vagus nerve stimulator. In July 2016, Dr. Tracey and colleagues published their research in the Proceedings of the National Academy of Sciences. They showed a significant reduction in rheumatoid arthritis symptoms and tumor necrosis factor (a marker of inflammation) in 28 patients with varying degrees of the disease. This was as a result of implanting an electrical vagus nerve stimulator.

In another study, Dr. Natelson and colleagues found that implanting a vagus nerve stimulator in fibromyalgia patients resulted in significant clinical improvements. After 11 months, seven of the patients improved dramatically and five patients no longer qualified for a fibromyalgia diagnosis, which was quite an outstanding outcome. Dr. Natelson said he had never seen a result like this with any other fibromyalgia treatment. The important thing to keep in mind is that you do not need an electrical implant to have that sort of effect on your vagus nerve. There are numerous very simple and free ways of improving your vagus nerve function. We will talk about those strategies shortly.

Cell Danger Response

What I also want to put on your radar is a phenomenon called the cell danger response (CDR), which I mentioned very briefly in the Introduction. If you are interested in exploring this in more detail, you can follow I just want to highlight here the link between the CDR and the vagus nerve. This is relevant to anybody suffering with chronic fatigue but also other diseases, including autoimmune diseases. The CDR is a natural process by which our mitochondria protect and defend themselves from threats such as infections, toxins, physical and psychological trauma, and other environmental stressors. The CDR is also a healthy way our bodies heal after injury.

However, when the CDR is chronically activated, the coordination between the two limbs of the vagus nerve is disrupted.

The ventral vagus nerve is no longer able to inhibit the survival responses, which now start to dominate. What this means for mitochondrial function is that if the CDR is activated, our mitochondria cannot maintain this defensive mode and maintain energy production at the normal level at the same time. So with chronically activated CDR, mitochondrial function will be compromised. That is when people experience chronic-fatigue related symptoms. Even though there are many factors affecting mitochondrial function, addressing your vagal tone will have a positive impact on the ability of your cells to produce energy.

Strategies That Increase Vagal Tone, Deepen the Mind-Body Connection & Balance the Brain

We are now going to focus on strategies to improve vagal tone. We will discuss different approaches to vagus nerve stimulation, what to do, as well as what not to do, and how to make vagus nerve work part of your daily routine.

Stimulating the Vagus Nerve

One way of dividing the vagus nerve activating techniques is into "bottom-up" and "top-down" approaches. Below is a list, but this is not exhaustive in any way. I am sure you can add to it yourself.

Top-Down Approaches

Top-down treatments strengthen the ability of the upper brain, the neocortex, to monitor your body's reactions and then step back and modulate the reactions of the amygdala. They include:

- Meditation/mindfulness
- Havening Techniques/EFT/EMDR/Somatic Experiencing
- Psychotherapy
- Positive social connection
- Expressing gratitude
- Laughter
- Prayer
- Bach flower remedies
- Connecting to nature.

Bottom-Up Approaches

These approaches help us act positively on the vagus nerve via affecting the body. They include:

- Deep breathing
- Singing/chanting/drumming/listening to music
- Yoga/tai chi/qigong/Feldenkreis/dance/walking/exercise in general
- Massage
- Craniosacral therapy
- Biofeedback
- Acupressure/acupuncture/auricular acupuncture
- Essential oils
- Coffee enemas
- Colon hydrotherapy
- Gargling / gag reflex
- Cold showers
- Fasting
- Sleeping on your side
- Probiotics/EFAs/vitamin D
- Sun exposure
- Sauna therapy

- Bubble baths
- Frequency-specific microcurrent therapy
- PEMF therapy
- Different vagus nerve stimulation devices.

Direct vs. Indirect Vagus Nerve Conditioning

We can also talk about vagus nerve stimulation in terms of its direct and indirect effects. It is very important to distinguish between those approaches. When you do Havening® or meditation, for example, you are soothing the nervous system. With these modalities you actually activate the ventral vagus nerve directly. That is one way of making your vagus nerve stronger. You activate it directly time and time again, and it becomes more responsive over time. But that is not the only way. We can also train the nervous system response through positive adaptations, which is just as powerful but not suitable for everybody right away.

In this case, we actually put ourselves under stress temporarily and then immediately return to the relaxation response when the stressor is removed. So rather than activate the ventral vagus nerve directly, we stimulate the sympathetic fight-or-flight response. However, because this is done in a controlled way, it is not harmful. It is the opposite. This allows for our mind and body to adapt. So then when stress comes along, we can withstand it because we have made ourselves more resilient. This is what we classify as good stress.

We are talking about hormesis here. Hormesis is a phenomenon of dose-response relationships, in which something that can produce potentially undesirable biological effects at high doses may produce beneficial or adaptive effects at low doses. One example of this is exercise. If we dose exercise appropriately, the body adapts without getting overwhelmed. We become stronger and healthier as a result. It is the same with cold therapy or heat therapy. If you spend all day in the sauna, it will not be good for you, but you can build up your tolerance.

Another example is breathing. Some people think that all breathing techniques are about relaxation. That is not true. Wim Hof breathing, if you are familiar with it, or the Breath of Fire, are stress-based breathing techniques. Do they work? Absolutely! But they might not be for everyone right away. Deep, slow breathing on the other hand, particularly when we really elongate the exhale, is a relaxation technique that activates the vagus nerve directly. So this is just something to keep in mind. Ideally, I recommend using a mixture of both. You want to get as much variety when it comes to increasing vagal tone as possible. Just like we need a varied food diet, we need a varied vagus nerve "diet."

The reason I am highlighting the difference between those two approaches is that if somebody has unresolved trauma and/or their nervous system is very sensitive, they may not respond well to those hormetic vagus nerve stimulation methods. In those cases, if the body is stressed even temporarily, this may be emotionally or physically triggering and overwhelming. Even a cold shower or gargling may be too much. This will improve as the nervous system is being rebalanced, but until then, only techniques that have a calming effect should be used. This is why you should always listen to your body when trying these different approaches.

Having the Correct Expectations

In order to have a meaningful impact on your health, vagus nerve activation needs to become part of your daily routine.

This is not the kind of thing that you do once or twice and then forget about it. You will need to make some of these techniques that achieve parasympathetic activation habitual to be able to recondition your nervous system. Nervous system dysregulation is created over time; it is the same with reconditioning.

Before we continue, I want pause for a moment and make sure that we set the right expectations for this work. You will see people online saying: *Just do some cold showers or gargling to stimulate your vagus nerve.* Often this sounds like it is so simple. The reality is quite different. Just to be clear: vagus nerve stimulation is not only helpful but essential. It helps you stabilize your nervous system and build some neurological resilience. However, if you have those emotional symptoms we have discussed previously, which basically means unresolved trauma, attachment issues, and limiting beliefs about yourself and the world, then you would need to be doing vagus nerve stimulation around the clock to fully recondition your nervous system. This is because that unresolved background emotional toxicity will continuously stimulate your fight, flight, or even freeze response.

Let us assume you do some breathing exercises, and maybe you even do some yoga or meditation, but you spend the rest of your day activating fight, flight, or freeze, for whatever reason. In this case, you could still be spending around 80 to 90 percent of your day in survival states. This is actually quite common. If that is the case, you will still perpetuate any disease state that you may already be in, and you might not even be able to prevent your health from deteriorating. Those techniques will still help you feel better in that moment, but if 80 to 90 percent of your time is spent feeling unworthy, undeserving, anxious, depressed, worrying about the future, being negative, beating yourself up about things you should do better, trying to control everything in your environment, and so on, activating your ventral vagus for 10 to 20 percent of the time is not going to be enough to make you healthy.

Plus, remember that in addition to those emotional aspects that people are often not even aware of, if you eat foods that you are sensitive to, or you are exposed to chemical toxins, EMFs, etc., this also adds to the stress load.

So yes, vagus nerve stimulation is great, and we can use it to exercise the ventral vagus nerve like we do muscles in the gym, which helps us rebalance our nervous system, but if we do not address the underlying causes of this dysfunction, simple vagus nerve stimulation is not going to be enough to achieve optimal health.

So again, you cannot shortcut those things. Some people always want to biohack everything, but we need to do this work properly to experience the real transformations that I know people can experience. You cannot gargle your way out of trauma and into health! It is ridiculous to even suggest that. So to summarize this point, vagus nerve stimulation is an essential part of my method because it is a great tool that helps us with reconditioning of the nervous system, but it is only one part of my method for the reasons I have just discussed. It will get you some of the way if you are trying to heal from chronic health symptoms, but on its own it is not going to be sufficient if the root causes of your nervous system dysregulation are not addressed.

How to Build Vagus Nerve Stimulation into Your Life

What I suggest for you to start with is to commit to a few weeks where you do your chosen exercises every day. You prioritize them and make them happen. I would say commit to at least four weeks of daily vagus nerve stimulation to begin with. If you do that, you should start to feel some positive impact, which then will encourage you to continue.

If for some reason you do not feel any positive impact, it is likely because you are extremely emotionally toxic and spend the majority of your waking hours (and even during sleep) in the fight, flight, or freeze response. If that is the case, you have a few options. You either continue with the vagus nerve stimulation exercises, increasing their frequency and duration, hoping that eventually you will tip that balance and start to feel the positive benefits of your vagus nerve work, or you continue with the vagus nerve exercises while also implementing the other steps of my method for a more holistic approach to your healing.

So How Do You Know You Have Started to Recondition Your Nervous System?

You know that something is improving when your response to everyday stressors changes and you do not get triggered in the way you used to. You also notice that when something stressful takes place, you can drop more easily back into the ventral vagus response once the stressor is gone. In other words, you are able to bring yourself back into a calm state more easily, which is supposed to be your baseline. In those first few weeks of doing the vagus nerve work, you have an opportunity to fine tune what works best for you. You then need to continue to make sure you can enjoy long-lasting benefits of having a strong, responsive vagus nerve. This by the way is only possible if you make this sustainable for yourself. So you need to figure out a little routine that is sustainable. That is key.

In addition, please remember that it is more impactful to activate your vagus nerve as frequently as possible for shorter periods of time than do a relaxing activity for a longer period but less frequently. You will recondition your nervous system more quickly if you do that. So frequency is more important than duration. You should also get in the habit of building awareness of what state you are in at any given time. So as frequently as you can, stop and ask yourself: *Am I in the rest-digest-detoxify-heal response right now, or am I in fight, flight, or freeze?* Keep bringing yourself back to the ventral vagus response whenever you catch yourself in fight, flight, or freeze. Just remember that you are either completely relaxed and safe or you are not, in which case the stress response is triggered. Unless this is good stress that helps you adapt, you should attempt to switch to the relaxation response.

So in terms of what is more effective, it is better to choose to gargle twice a day after cleaning your teeth, and set yourself reminders to do 2-3 minutes of deep breathing throughout the day (for example, before a meal) than it is to try to meditate for an hour. This is not to say that meditating for an hour is not effective or that it will not make you more resilient. If you can do that regularly and effectively, it will. However, this is not a reasonable expectation for many people, particularly at the beginning. So as you are shortlisting those vagus nerve stimulating activities that are most appealing to you, which is very important for sustainability, think about how you will incorporate them into your daily routine. I have already given an example of combining gargling with teeth cleaning. Other examples include doing an activity upon waking up or just before going to sleep, e.g., a few minutes of deep breathing, Havening®, or gratitude practice. I encourage you to spend some time thinking about setting your new routine up because that will make the implementation much easier. After a while, it will just be something you do.

What Not to Do & What to Be Aware of When Doing Vagus Nerve Work

When it comes to addressing the nervous system dysregulation and improving your vagal tone, it is not just about what you do. IT IS JUST AS MUCH ABOUT WHAT YOU DON'T DO. This goes back to what I said before. It is really about how much time overall you spend in the relaxation versus the stress response, as that impacts how your nervous system is conditioned. Even though most people's poor vagal tone has its origins in childhood trauma and even intergenerational trauma, many people make it much worse for themselves with the everyday conscious choices they make, such as watching mainstream news.

It is time for some straight talk again. Basically, you really are not going to be able to have a healing effect on your nervous system, no matter how many vagus nerve activation exercises you do, if you expose yourself to garbage and program your mind negatively on a daily basis. Below are some things you should avoid if you want to have a good vagus nerve function.

Watching & Reading Mainstream News

This also includes other doom and gloom media output. When you watch mainstream news, you are subject to very sophisticated methods of mind control that are designed to instill fear and make you feel like a caged animal. They do it with language, images, tonality, symbolism, and special frequencies. You may have some cognitive dissonance reading this, but I guarantee that this is, unfortunately, true. Regardless how resistant you think you are to this, if you watch mainstream news regularly, your subconscious is gradually being programmed with messages that you really do not want as part of your belief system.

You then create your reality based on that programming. So I recommend you cut it out of your life or, at the very least, be very discerning and minimize your exposure.

Spending Too Much Time on Social Media

Social media platforms, are mostly toxic and divisive, and are very much used to control public opinion. This was what Fakebook was originally designed for. Again, if you do not think this is factual information, do your own research. In addition, there are studies to show that spending too much time on social media makes people dumber and more insecure. It is all cleverly designed to be addictive. It sucks you in, and before you know it, you have wasted another hour of your life, or two, or ten. No matter how good you want to make it, it always ends up toxic in some way. So unless all you have on your timeline is fluffy kittens, I recommend drastically reducing the time you spend engaging with it.

Watching Violent Movies or Movies That Produce a Fearful or Angry Response

The same goes for books or computer games. Remember that your nervous system does not distinguish if you are feeling fearful because of a real-life situation or something that you see on a TV screen. It responds the same way.

Surrounding Yourself with Toxic People

By toxic people I mean people who are negative, put you down, or with whom you do not feel safe or good about yourself. This may be harder in some cases, but it has to be done, and healthy boundaries have to be set. You will find this challenging if you have poor self-worth. By the way, becoming more aware and avoiding negative input does not mean you disconnect from reality altogether. It just means making better choices so that you are not constantly undoing the work you are putting in. Ask yourself if you really need to have conversations with people about all the bad stuff that they think might happen, for example. How does that serve you? How does that help you be healthy? It does not. Plus, you create your reality with your thoughts every single minute of every single day. In the quantum field there are multiple timelines, and you are the one who decides which timeline you are going to end up on based on the thoughts you have. So when you surround yourself with negative influences from whatever sources, you are going to be influenced by them and create your reality based on that.

Talking to Yourself in a Negative Way

Most people are completely unaware of their negative self-talk, but it is very important to become more conscious of what you are saying to yourself. From now on, I recommend you start paying more attention to it, and every time you catch yourself thinking anything negative or self-critical, I want you to use my SCC method. This stands for STOP – CHANGE STATE – COUNTER. First, as you aware of a negative thought, stop. Then immediately change state. This should ideally be something physical (e.g., jumping a few times on the spot or waving your arms in the air). If you are unable to perform a physical task, you can imagine you are doing it. You can also sing or hum a tune or solve a quick mathematical problem in your head (e.g., 48 + 56). This will interrupt the program you are running at this point and will put your brain on a different track. Then, you counter the negative thought with something positive.

For example, if your original destructive thought was: *Why did I do that? I am such a loser!*, you can counter it with saying: *I did my best and I choose to accept my best as good enough.* If you do not interrupt that original negative thought, you will create a negative feeling. That will then create more negative thoughts, which will create more negative feelings, and you will get on that negative loop, which activates fight or flight. Even though we need to rewire those programs at the subconscious level, it is also important to consciously start interrupting negative thought patterns. So please start doing this straight away. Most of the time, you do not even know you are doing it, so you need to become more conscious, and over time, you will get better at it.

Eating When Stressed

If you eat in a stressed state, you do not digest food properly, and that leads to digestive system dysfunction that further contributes to poor vagal tone. It is also a shortcut to developing food sensitivities. Keep in mind that even reading emails or watching TV can put you in the stress response. Not to mention eating on the go. You need to put emphasis on eating slowly and chewing properly. I recommend that before you eat, if you do not already do this, express gratitude for what you are about to eat. Expressing gratitude activates the rest-and-digest response.

Resonance

Another very important thing is to only go with what resonates with you. There are many ways to stimulate your vagus nerve, so do not feel that you need to torture yourself with something you really dislike. Just because something has a potential to stimulate the vagus nerve, does not mean it is right for you. THIS IS IMPORTANT! If performing a task is causing you anxiety or you have some sort of a negative response to it for whatever reason, this will actually put you in the fight-or-flight mode, and the result might actually be the opposite to what you intended.

Take, for example, seated meditation. That is a great tool to stimulate the vagus nerve, but it is NOT for everybody. There are many people who are not at a point in their life, for whatever reason, where they can benefit from seated meditation. They will come away from it more wound-up and irritated than they were before they started. If that is the case, if that is your experience, you are not achieving vagus nerve activation with this particular modality. I encourage you to look into why that is, as there is always a reason, but the bottom line is, you need to do something else to stimulate your vagus nerve until you have resolved this.

Another good example is social connection. Just because social interaction has the potential to stimulate the vagus nerve does not mean it will have that effect on everybody. If somebody has social anxiety, then social interaction will be stressful. This, again, will have a root cause that I suggest should be looked into. It is the same with being in nature. Personally, I find being close to nature one of the most relaxing and regenerating activities. However, if somebody has a phobia or fear of insects, for example, which again can be easily addressed, they might be on edge the entire time they are out in nature. In this case, they will not achieve vagus nerve activation. That underlying low-level anxiety will be further conditioning their already overactive stress response.

So to summarize, in order to have a positive impact on your nervous system, you need to have this *ooh, this is so nice* or *this is relaxing* feeling. Naturally, when you use those hormetic methods, you may not always enjoy the associated discomfort as you are doing the activity, for example, when you feel the muscles burning during exercise, when you are standing under a cold shower, or when you are getting really hot in a sauna. But as long as you feel good afterwards, it will work well. So choose vagus nerve activation activities based on what makes you feel good and what you enjoy. Before we move on, I want to invite you to join me for a breathing exercise. This particular breathing technique is a great way to activate your vagus nerve, so see if this resonates with you. You can find the video in the Additional Resources. I have also included another video you may like that combines breathing with movement.

Measuring Vagal Tone

Some people like to measure where they are and what progress they are making. Is it essential? No. When you increase your vagal tone, you notice. Everything functions better, and you are more relaxed and more resilient, which means you can get over stressful experiences more quickly. In addition, your brain is sharper, your digestion is more efficient, any supplements that you take have more of an effect, and your immune system is better balanced. That is more than enough for some people, and they do not need numbers to prove to them that their commitment to vagus nerve work is benefiting them.

You can use journaling to note the differences in the way you feel. This is a great awareness building exercise because when you are journaling and writing how you feel, it encourages you to be more aware. Additionally, if you look for positive changes and improvements, you will be reconditioning your nervous system to look for and focus on positives.

However, those who would like to measure how their vagal tone is improving can satisfy their curiosity by measuring heart rate variability (HRV). This is the best way of measuring vagal tone that we have. Please note that this is NOT the same as heart rate (HR). HRV measures time between consecutive heartbeats (in milliseconds), whereas your HR simply tells you how many times your heart beats per minute (bpm). We want our resting HR to be low (50 – 70 bpm), but we want our HRV to be high. Nope, this is not a mistake. You want your HRV to be high because you do not actually want your heart to beat like a metronome.

The normal variability in HR is due to the synergistic action of the two branches of the autonomic nervous system. The sympathetic nerves accelerate HR, while the parasympathetic response (the ventral vagus nerve) slows it down. This constant interaction is designed to maintain cardiovascular activity in its optimal range. The higher our HRV, the more variability in the way our heart beats. This is what we want, as this means our system is more adaptable compared to somebody whose heart beats in a more of a metronome fashion. Monotonously regular rhythm is actually bad news for your health and longevity. In addition to informing us about the health of our vagus nerve, HRV is one of the best predictors of mortality from all known causes of death.

There are many tools to measure HRV. If you are interested in learning more about HRV and how to measure it, look up the HeartMath Institute. They have tools you can purchase to help guide you through specific exercises. You can also learn about the concept of cardiac coherence, which is another important aspect of disease prevention and promoting health. Alternatively, there are a number of devices on the market that you can use to measure HRV. One I definitely do NOT recommend for this purpose is Fitbit. You can also use a HR monitor that is compatible with an HRV app you download on your phone.

Importance of Managing Day-to-Day Stress

Managing your day-to-day stress is, again, something that calls for you to be more consciously aware of what you are experiencing. Why is this important? Because day-to-day stress, even at low levels, tends to creep up on you. If you drift through every day unaware of your triggers and responses, and without counteracting stress, your mind and nervous system will be degraded over time. You may not actually notice the symptoms of that right away. You might think that you are not that affected by those low-grade everyday stressors, or you may simply be desensitized to some of them. Either way, if you do not counteract them on a regular basis, as they occur, your vagal tone will deteriorate over time.

This is another reason why I recommend you have a range of vagus nerve stimulation techniques that you use daily and that you become more aware about keeping your mind free of toxic influences. That way, you will be bringing more balance to your nervous system and you will be able to stop any stress from building up and causing further nervous system dysregulation. I always highly recommend that you immediately counter any traumatic experiences that may come your way with the different tools and techniques I am offering throughout this book. The reality is that life will always happen. You cannot prevent it but you can build your toolkit and counter any negative experiences as they arise to stop them from encoding neurologically.

Furthermore, stress kills brain cells and can even reduce the size of the brain. For example, persistent exposure to stress hormones and resulting inflammation reduces the hippocampus, which is part of the brain associated with memory and learning. Chronic stress ultimately also changes the neurochemicals in the brain, which modulate cognition and mood, including serotonin. Stress can also interfere with our balance between rational thinking and emotions. In fact, one of the signs that somebody's vagus nerve function is poor is their disproportionate reactions to everyday stresses and situations.

People whose ventral vagus nerve does not function well have a skewed perception of the world and people around them. They misinterpret what other people are trying to communicate and they tend to assume the worst. They wind themselves up very easily, tend to be very reactive, and jump to conclusions, which will have a negative impact on their self-worth and their relationships. Their brains say: *danger is everywhere*. On the other hand, a healthy ventral vagus nerve allows us to tap into our feelings that warn us of safety versus danger, to connect to ourselves and the world, and to empathize and bond with others, which supports safety. It also enables us to read other people's facial expressions and assess whether they are safe to approach or whether they should be avoided.

Connecting the Mind to the Body

This section of the book will be particularly important to you if you are currently challenged by accessing what your body is experiencing. I will repeat this over and over: *you must feel in order to heal.* What that means is that you have to be able to fully connect to your body in order to become healthy. If you are currently a bit of a floating head, meaning you live so

178

much in your head that you are not very aware of what goes on in the body, you need to address this disconnect in order to move forward in your healing process. You should know that this is one reason why you have bodily symptoms. It is because your body says: *I will make you come out of your head. Here is some pain* (or whatever other symptom). Bodily symptoms are the body's way of making you pay attention to the body in the hope that you are going to give the body what it needs. Just to clarify, even if you are good at connecting to the body, in a sense that you feel emotions and you can identify what you feel, those bodily sensations mean there is unresolved trauma that is sitting in the tissues and your energy field.

Unfortunately, many people out there are disconnected from their bodies due to early trauma and they only feel their bodies when the body makes them, so to speak. Attachment and other trauma that causes people to disconnect from their body sets them up for chronic illness. As the body is ignored, the symptoms get louder. As we know, the reason animals do not get traumatized in the way people do is because they do not hold on to emotional energy. They shake it off following, for example, being chased by another animal. We need to release that emotional energy trapped in our bodies, but that cannot be done when you do not allow yourself to connect with it. We want our minds and bodies to be connected and working in harmony. The following strategies I am going to share with you will help you do just that.

I know that when you are not entirely comfortable with something, or you feel like you are not good at something, there is this tendency to dodge it altogether, but I am urging you to push through this. Otherwise, you will not be able to heal your emotional toxicity or fully heal your body at the physical level.

179

It may help you to use some specific affirmations when doing this work, such as:

It is OK for me to feel.

It is safe for me to feel.

I choose to feel so I can heal.

I choose to feel so I can resolve my blocks and traumas.

In addition, if when doing the exercises you start to feel overwhelmed in any way, here is what I want you to do:

1. Start applying Havening Touch®, meaning you immediately start stroking your face, your arms, or your hands in the way I have already taught you.

2. Slow your breathing down while you allow yourself to feel what you are feeling without judgment or attachment. In this case, attachment means resistance. If you start saying: *I don't want to feel this, I don't want to feel this* - that is resistance. As we already said, if you resist, the emotion will persist. Plus, remember that your subconscious does not understand negation, so if you keep saying you do not want to be feeling something, you will feel it even more.

3. While you are stroking your arms, bring to your mind a memory of when you felt safe, or someone, something, or some activity that makes you feel safe. The emotion will subside within a few minutes. It usually is quite quick, unless you resist it, so just let it be, breathe slowly, and haven. You can also affirm: *I am safe. I am OK.*

4. Alternatively, if your mind starts going towards negative thoughts, you can use the SCC method I have taught you previously.

Now that you have these strategies, you can engage with the exercises fully, knowing that it is safe for you to do so. If you experience a lot of dissociation due to trauma, when you do these exercises, you start to feel more present. You might start to notice more things in your environment. You may notice colors to be brighter. If you have been in shutdown mode for a long time, you may briefly experience fight-or-flight when you start to reconnect with your body. This may be new but should not last. It actually means that the energy in the system is starting to shift in a positive way. That said, if you feel it is too much, use the tools I have given you to calm yourself down.

Slowing Everything Down Exercise

This is a very gentle exercise to get you started. You perform these movements every day, but you move through them quickly. What we are going to do here is slow everything down. So first, take a couple of deeper breaths and connect with gravity. Notice where your body is in contact with solid surfaces, such as the surface you are sitting on, as well as the floor. Connect with this sense of *weighted-ness* in your hips and your feet, that feeling of grounding. As you are feeling that, allow everything to slow down. Now, look straight ahead and then move your head gently and slowly to the right. Then slowly look up and down. Now, slowly move you head to the left and look up and down. Then again to the right.

So basically, you are just very slowly looking around, slowing yourself right down. As you are doing that, see if you can pause on something that catches your eye, that you think is interesting in some way. Allow yourself to take that in. Notice every detail. Notice now how your body is feeling as you are slowly looking around, examining your surroundings. Notice any sensations or emotions that may come up as you are taking in what you are looking at. Now close your eyes and just hear what you hear. Again, move your head gently around and just listen. What can you hear? If there are many different sounds, try to pick out one and focus on it for a moment. Maybe your surroundings are fairly silent, but what about those subtle sounds? Like the sound of your breathing? Just focus on it for a moment and notice any bodily sensations associated with that sound or sounds.

Feeling for Contrasting Sensations

Focusing on contrasting sensations is a great way to reconnect your head back to your body.

First, take a few cleansing breaths. Make them deep and slow. Close your eyes. Adjust your body position so that your shoulders are back and down and your chest is open. Now think of somebody you dislike. This can be anybody: a family member, a neighbor, maybe a co-worker. Bring this person to mind and think about why you dislike them first. What is it about them that makes you dislike them? What is it specifically that they do or say? Perhaps, it is the way they say it that triggers you and makes you dislike them. Now feel for any sensations in your body. Where in your body is the sensation associated with disliking this person? It is not in your head. If you think you feel this in your head, it is your ego trying to interfere with the exercise, so get out of your head and connect to the body. Where is the sensation in your body when you think about this person? What is it specifically that they do or say, or what they may have done or said in the past, that makes you dislike them? Describe that sensation of disliking them. Where is it in the body? What is the temperature or texture of that feeling?

Sit with it for a moment. Accept it for what it is. Let go of any attachment. Just observe it.

Now clear you mind and take a few deep breaths. Breathe in through your nose if possible and very slowly exhale through your mouth. Now somebody you love to your mind—a person close to your heart or maybe an animal. Imagine them clearly. Now pay attention to the body. How is the body responding this time? What sensations can you feel? What emotion or emotions? What is it specifically about this person or animal that makes you feel this way? What do they do to make you feel the way you do towards them? Where is the emotion in your body? Connect with this emotion. Let yourself experience it fully. Now consider how differently this feels from what you felt a moment ago. Consider the contrast. If you would like to follow my instructions, please go to the Additional Resources for this exercise.

Another exercise that you can do to help you feel contrasting sensations involves using essential oils. For this exercise you will need two different essential oils (or other scents): one that you are not so keen on and one you really like. First, close your eyes and take a few deeper breaths. Smell the oil you are not so keen on. What is it about this scent that you dislike? Drop into the body to examine what sensations you are experiencing as a result of connecting with this particular scent. Notice all the bodily responses you are having. Perhaps this smell reminds you of something. Spend a few minutes tuning into your body and how it feels. Now, smell the oil you really like. Again, notice how your body is responding. Notice all the subtleties and differences in the way your body is feeling now. Spend a few minutes connecting with the sensations and noticing the contrast in how your body has responded to those two scents.

I recommend that you do the same exercise with taste. Close your eyes and take a few deep breaths before you start. Take something into your mouth that you are not so keen on and focus entirely on the bite inside your mouth. Give it your full attention for a couple of minutes and then, once you swallow that bite, connect with the bodily sensations that it created. Follow that with something that you particularly like and observe the contrasting sensations. It is important to slow everything down and focus your full attention on this one activity.

If you found those exercises easy, that means your connection between your head and your body is reasonably good. Still, that was great training for you, as you can never have too much awareness of your body. If these exercises challenged you in any way, I suggest you repeat them until you are able to drop into your body and connect with your bodily sensations easily. Make sure that you feel safe in your surroundings when you are doing any of this work. If you feel jumpy in your environment, your brain will be on red alert and will not let you engage properly.

Balancing the Brain

I also want to encourage you to incorporate specific exercises to balance your brain so you have more harmony between the two hemispheres. Why is that important? Because having an organized brain creates a vastly different experience of the world compared to having a disorganized brain. Some of the signs of your hemispheres being out of balance and you having a disorganized brain include:

- depleted mental energy
- lack of motivation

- difficulty concentrating due to decreased ability to filter out distracting information (this is often a key reason why people are not able to meditate)
- negative OCD loops, as well as ADHD and similar labels, are a sign of a disorganized brain
- anxiety
- rigid thinking (lacking that behavioral flexibility that is essential if you want to be resilient)
- problems with intimacy
- poor cognitive function, memory issues
- difficulty processing sensory input (e.g., heightened sensitivity to light, sound, etc.).

In contrast, somebody with an organized brain:
- has no issues with mental energy, which means they can maintain their concentration for long periods
- can filter out distractions so they can study or meditate effectively
- can develop new skills easily because they have efficient pathways to all parts of the brain
- has good short- and long-term memory
- is good at extrapolating information and drawing conclusions
- has no issues with verbal expression and communicating with others
- tends to be more creative and more excited about life
- is good at interpreting emotional responses
- is flexible and adaptable (they do not have the need to control every little detail of their life).

So What Is the Process of Getting the Brain More Balanced?

Step one is to calm down the nervous system. By reducing stress and calming the nervous system, we are preparing the brain for deep and lasting change. Overactive sympathetic and dorsal responses drain neural energy. We need ventral vagus function to be good in order to restore that energy. So this is another reason to put work into improving your vagal tone and your emotional regulation. Once neurologically safe and stable, we can start reorganizing the brain with vestibulary input. This will further help to prevent getting stuck in those shutdown or hyper-arousal states.

Below are some of the best vestibular activation exercises I recommend. These exercises will help you improve your brain organization and build neurological resilience.

Stabilizing Your Gaze

Look straight ahead. Now turn your head to the right while keeping your eyes facing forward. Make sure you are not fully turning your head—just a 45-degree angle. Then turn your head towards the left at the same angle. Aim to perform this exercise 10 times and repeat throughout the day.

Vertical & Horizontal Head Movement

Move your head from the left to the right slowly. Repeat 10 to 20 times but keep increasing the pace gradually until the maximum comfortable speed has been reached. Stop for 10 seconds. Restart the procedure again. Then, repeat the process, moving your head up and down.

Walking on Uneven Terrain

Orientating in Space

Jump up and then pause when you land to allow your brain to work out your positioning in space. Always keep your knees soft.

Balance Training

Balancing the body helps you balance the brain. There are many different balance exercises you can do, for example, balancing on one leg. You should be able to stand on one leg without falling over for at least a minute. When this becomes easy, try it with your eyes closed. You should be able to do this comfortably for at least 30 to 60 seconds. If you are not able to, this means your brain hemispheres are not very well balanced. If you practice this regularly, you will improve quite quickly. This work tends to be very rewarding. When you are doing this exercise, make sure that you are close to a wall that you can use for support so you do not hurt yourself.

Yoga & Pilates

Perform Tasks with Your Non-dominant Hand or Foot
This can be teeth brushing, hair brushing, even writing. Pick a couple of activities that you do every day anyway so you do not have to spend any extra time doing it. You will, of course, be slower but again, this will improve.

Perform Cognitive Tasks That You Are Not Very Good at
Things such as learning new language, doing puzzles, crosswords, Sudoku, etc. obviously help the brain. But the key point here is that if you are good at language type exercises like

crosswords, do not just do more of that, which is what most people do. You should push yourself to do the opposite if you want to develop your brain. Pick something you really suck at and do that. If you suck at numbers, do more of that. Doing what you are already good at is not as effective at building your neurology as doing things that challenge you.

Reorganize Your Brain with Sound

You may have heard of binaural beats. There are also other types of beats, such as monaural and isochronic beats, which are great for brain entrainment. I always use specific frequencies in my meditations depending on what I am trying to achieve. It makes sense to me to combine those different strategies to rewire the nervous system and the brain in almost efficient way.

In summary, you have many different options to rebalance your brain and your autonomic nervous system. When you do these exercises regularly, you build new neural connections and you improve your brain organization, which means more resilience, better cognitive function, and more mental energy. You can then further develop this until your brain, nervous system function, and your brain balance is optimal for you.

Action Points

1. Design your vagus nerve stimulation routine by choosing activities that resonate with you from the list I have provided in this chapter. You can also use Affirmational Havening® and Future Outcome Havening®, which I introduced you to in Chapter 1, for this purpose. I am providing you with some additional practical videos, including Gratitude Havening®, as well as specific breathing and movement exercises in the Additional Resources (https://www.dr-eva.com/shs-resources).

2. Start using my SCC method to counter negative self-talk.

3. Choose one or two brain balancing exercises and perform them daily.

Understanding & Mastering Emotions

Recognizing Core & Complex Emotions

John came to see me because he had started having problems sleeping and as a result of not sleeping properly, his health started to break down. He started experiencing gut issues, constant headaches, and muscular aches. He was very anxious, impatient with others, and was unable to maintain his concentration for more than 15 minutes at a time. On the surface, his anxiety was not specific to anything. He was just extremely worried about his future, and the more worried he was, the worse his physical symptoms were getting, which was further feeding his anxiety. This is a common vicious cycle many people find themselves caught up in.

Unsurprisingly, upon some examination, his doctor concluded that he must have developed generalized anxiety disorder and offered him drugs. What about trying to discover where this came from? Uncovering the root cause? Never mind. Just numb yourself with some drugs and get on with it. But John was not interested in just popping medication and, unlike his doctor, he decided to get to the bottom of what he was experiencing. Within a couple of minutes of our initial conversation, it was obvious to me that his insomnia had a psychological trigger. It was also obvious to me that John was one of these people who have become very emotionally muddled. He kept saying: *I am just worried about everything all the time.* He was not able to tell what he was feeling and why. It had all blended into this one feeling of anxiety. But of course, anxiety is only a label. The core emotion behind anxiety is fear. So the question was, what triggered the feeling of fear, and what event in his life had got neurologically encoded in such a way as to produce his generalized anxiety?

What was curious about John's case was that his insomnia started shortly after his 49th birthday. Thorough questioning did not reveal any events in the 12 to 18 months prior. There had not been any change in his circumstances or any significant experiences during that time. It was as though somebody flipped a switch in his mind. We looked at the different triggers that made him anxious, and the common theme revolved around not being able to cope, fend for himself, and provide for his family. So what makes somebody go from functioning well to being a blabbering mess in a matter of weeks if nothing had changed in their circumstances?Early trauma.

As we dug deeper, it transpired that John had had a knee surgery when he was nine years old. It was not a major surgery, but John remembered the surgeon saying to his mother that the knee should hold up until he was 50, probably meaning that John may at some point have some aches or might have to avoid straining the joint. But to little John, this sounded ominous, and it did frighten him. He remembered wondering at that time what was going to happen to him after he turned 50. How was he going to cope without a functioning knee? His mind got carried away, as is frequently the case with traumatic encoding, and generalized this to him not being able to cope, work, or have a normal life. This fear had been dormant in his subconscious until he turned 49 years old.

At this point, his subconscious mind got triggered and flipped. It started running this program that went something like this: *The next stop is 50. That is when you were told by the surgeon your knee would be done. Your whole life is soon going to change, and you will not be able to cope.* This produced anxiety that started dominating John's life. He felt like he was running out of time, and yet at the same time, he was afraid to engage with life. This subconscious program was running on a loop. This stopped him from sleeping, which further exacerbated his heightened emotional state. Once we figured out the connection, it took one session to clear that trauma and put John's subconscious on a different track. John started sleeping better almost right away.

He was delighted with the result, but the bigger lesson for him was to develop some emotional intelligence. By his own admission, he had never been that emotionally aware, so it was very difficult for him to recognize what he was feeling and why.

Even though he experienced different emotions—fear of not being in control, fear of loss, fear of being disabled, grief after the life he was going to lose, anger and shame about not being able to cope with his emotions, etc.—he was not aware of what he was feeling. He just wanted the feelings to go away, and the more he was trying to push them away, the more they overwhelmed him. After a while, it just became one thick cloud of anxiety. The interesting thing was that if John had been more emotionally aware, he would have probably figured the connection out himself, or at least he would not have tied himself in such an emotional knot. There is always a reason why we feel what we feel. When we become proficient in recognizing our emotional responses and triggers, there is no longer a need to be terrified or overwhelmed by what we feel. Particularly, when we have some great tools to help us discharge emotional energy.

Should Emotions Be Categorized into Good & Bad?

To be able to master emotions, we need to first understand them and understand their purpose. In other words, to have emotional immunity you first have to develop emotional intelligence. To begin with, I want to discuss this idea of emotions being good or bad. What do you think? Do you think emotions can be divided into good and bad?

Let me give you my viewpoint on this. It depends on the context. If we consider emotional states from the point of view of energy and consciousness, then we have to accept that there is no division into good or bad because in higher dimensional realms, nothing is good or bad; it just is. It is a concept called neutrality. Dividing anything into good and bad (duality) is the nature of living in our 3D physical reality. But even at the level of our 3D physical reality, whether emotions are good or bad depends on the context. It essentially comes down to chronic versus acute. Every emotion serves a purpose. All of them. Basically, emotions are messengers, and they also help us get from A to B in our lives.

Emotions are tools. They are not the cause of the discomfort; they are messengers designed to help us with the discomfort. This applies even to the emotions that people usually label as "bad," for example, fear, anger, sadness. They are there to help us. They push us to act, and escaping them is not productive. Emotions become negative if we do not understand them, or if we suppress them, deny them, or desensitize to them, yet experience them chronically. Sadness, for example, helps us let go. That is what grief is all about. Anger helps us set better boundaries. Fear helps us survive. It is there to activate fight-or-flight and save our skin when the situation calls for it. If we did not have fear, we would not have survived as a species. Those emotions also trigger growth. When we experience trauma and we experience fear, anger, etc., it is working through these emotions that then allows us to experience post-traumatic growth. So, in that sense, you cannot say they are negative.

The problem arises when our brain takes it too far; in other words, when everything is perceived as a threat, whether it is real or not. This is, as I said before, related to the nervous system being wired for fight-or-flight as a result of early exposure to stress and early trauma. When everything is perceived as a threat, then these emotions start to dominate. When they are experienced chronically, that is when they become negative because they imbalance our nervous systems and ruin our mental and physical health. Again, these emotions also become negative if we suppress them, resist them in some way, pretend they are not there, or try to escape them. That is because suppression, resistance, and escapism does not make them go away. They are still there, and that is when they become chronic and people often desensitize to them. If you desensitize and become better at ignoring them, it does not mean that they are not there, or they have been resolved. They are still being experienced chronically in the emotional, and then mental, and finally physical body.

Core Emotions

Let us now look at the different categories of emotions. That will help you recognize what you are really experiencing. Plus, when you have different labels coming to you, you can strip all that down and identify which basic emotion is really behind it. This will be super helpful to you because understanding what emotion you are feeling, and why, can take a sting out of an emotionally intense experience. There are a few different schools of thought when it comes to categorizing emotions, but I choose to break them down into six key classes of emotions: happiness, fear, anger, sadness, love, and disgust. Core emotions inform us about our environment. *Am I safe or in danger? What do I need or want? What do I not want? Am I sad? Am I hurt? What brings me pleasure? What disgusts me? What excites me?* Core emotions are hard-wired in our brains, which means they are not subject to conscious control. Each core emotion is pre-wired to set off certain physiological reactions that prepare us for an action, like running from danger. If we understand them and connect to them, core emotions give us important information and help us thrive.

Happiness

Most people are able to correctly identify when they feel happy. There are different reasons for people to feel this emotion, but usually, you may experience happiness if you are:

- close and connected to people you care about
- safe and secure
- doing something that triggers sensory pleasure
- absorbed in an activity
- relaxed and at peace.

Some words you can use to describe what you feel when you experience happiness include: contentment, amusement, joy, relief, pride, excitement, peace, calm, satisfaction, compassion, euphoria, ecstasy, bliss, elation, delight, jubilation, enthusiasm, exhilaration, pleasure, cheerfulness, zest, optimism, interest, triumph, and gratitude.

Fear

You feel fear when you sense any type of threat. It is usually visible in somebody's physiology. They may be sweating, their breathing rate may be elevated, etc. Depending on that perceived threat, fear can range from mild to severe. Fear can make you feel worried, doubtful, nervous, anxious, terrified, panicked, horrified, desperate, confused, stressed, apprehensive, overwhelmed, scared, frightened, on edge, out of control, uncertain, insecure, paranoid, phobic, threatened, mortified, trapped, uneasy, shocked, alarmed, terrorized, ambivalent, avoidant, or doubtful. When it comes to fear, it is also good to recognize the type of fear you are experiencing. We have some basic types of fear:

- fear of rejection/abandonment/criticism/not being accepted
- fear of not being in control/fear of change/fear of the unknown
- fear of failure/fear of success
- fear of intimacy/fear of commitment/fear of being vulnerable
- fear of adversity/hardship/illness/being in pain/death
- fear of loss (this could relate to freedom or whatever else that matters to you).

Your behavior and how you operate in life is going to be driven by one or more of those fears. For example, somebody who changes relationships like underwear may say they like to keep things "fresh," but what we are really dealing with here is a fear of commitment, or fear of being vulnerable. Somebody who tries to control everything in their environment is dominated by their fear of not being in control and fear of the unknown. Somebody who does things for other people, even though they do not really want to, and they moan about it afterwards, does those things because they fear being rejected (or not being accepted) or criticized. Somebody who does not want to try something new is very likely scared of not being good at it, underneath which is a fear of failure.

But what is even more interesting is that all fear is really about our survival being threatened and ultimately about fear of death. Fear often manifests as anger. Look at the Chaos 2020. People attacking others for not wearing masks, acting like complete animals at times, being very aggressive. All that we are dealing with here is those people's fear of death kicking in as a result of media programing. When people's brains are flooded with fear neurochemicals, they become reactive and lose the ability to see things for what they really are. So that is an obvious example. Let us now look at something at one that is not so obvious. Take a small thing that somebody finds irritating. Somebody said to me once that they felt irritated and triggered by their neighbors not mowing their lawn regularly enough. So I asked: *How is your neighbors not cutting their grass a problem for you? How is this threatening your survival?* Here is how the conversation went.

Because they're supposed to do it.

What happens if they don't?

They break the rules.
What happens when they break the rules?
Then other people may start breaking the rules too, since they
*   think they can get away with it.*
So what happens if everybody starts breaking the rules?
Then we will have anarchy!
What is the problem with that? How is anarchy a prob-
*   lem for you?*
Anarchy is a threat to my survival.

Do you understand? That is how your subconscious works. It connects everything to survival and produces emotional responses and behaviors to make sure you fend off the threat. That it is why it is so easy to plunge people into fear.

Anger

Anger usually happens when you experience some type of injustice or your boundaries get violated. This experience can make you feel threatened, trapped, and unable to defend yourself. Like I said, anger is connected to fear. It can also be linked to disgust. Many people think of anger as a negative thing, but it is a normal emotion that can help you know when a situation has become toxic and helps you set boundaries. Words you might use when you feel angry include: annoyed, frustrated, bitter, infuriated, irritated, mad, cheated, vengeful, insulted, agitated, enraged, hostile, aggressive, resentful, angst, and anguish. Some people may use stronger words, such as pissed off.

When somebody is openly angry, you can usually tell quite easily, but what about passive-aggressive behavior, which is basically sugar-coated hostility? Some signs of that include:

198

- denying being angry
- withdrawing or sulking
- provoking so that the other person expresses anger towards the person who is being passive aggressive
- agreeing to do something but purposely doing it below the acceptable standard
- making excuses for behaving badly when it is visible that the behavior is driven by resentment and hostility
- the person is incongruent: there is no alignment between what this person says, their behavior, and what they are feeling.

Sadness

Sadness is often experienced as a result of a loss. Remember that this does not just mean losing somebody. This can be a loss of anything related to the past, present, or future. For example, we can grieve over something that never happened (we never got to be something or do something in the past). We can also grieve over a relationship or a dream. When you are sad, you might describe yourself as lonely, heartbroken, gloomy, disappointed, hopeless, grieved, unhappy, lost, troubled, resigned, miserable, depressed, disinterested, alienated, homesick, humiliated, pitiful, suffering, nostalgic, apathetic, or in pain.

Disgust

You typically experience disgust as a reaction to unpleasant or unwanted situations. Similarly to anger, feelings of disgust can help to protect you from things you want to avoid. You can feel disgusted when you smell or taste something unpleasant. Poor hygiene, blood, rot, and death can trigger a disgust response

199

in some people. In this context, this may be the body's way of avoiding things that may carry transmittable diseases. But we can also experience moral disgust when we observe others engaging in behaviors that we find distasteful, immoral, or evil. And finally, many people have disgust towards themselves. Disgust might cause you to feel: dislike, revulsion, loathing, disapproval, aversion, offense, horror, uncomfortable, nauseated, disturbed, withdrawal, embarrassed, guilt, shame, hate, or contempt.

Love

This is the most powerful and most healing emotion. One of the highest in terms of vibrational frequency. It is important to feel it towards others and definitely towards yourself. Self-love is the pinnacle of healing. Feelings in this category include: feeling of oneness, intimacy, affection, longing, lust, fondness, attraction, adoration, sentimentality, admiration, appreciation, caring, arousal, desire, infatuation, passion, trusting, and acceptance.

Be Curious What Is Behind What You Are Feeling

So we have those basic categories of emotions and then I have given you many other words associated with each of them. We want to have an extensive vocabulary when it comes to emotions and we also want to be able to quickly identify which one of the main categories what we are feeling falls into. For example, we may feel disappointed. So what is behind that? It is sadness. We may feel anxious. It is important to realize that anxiety is really a fear of something. This helps us address what we are experiencing more efficiently, rather than go on a wild goose chase with something like anxiety, not realizing we are dealing with one of the key fears.

Now I would like you to spend a few minutes thinking through your day-to-day responses. I would like you to look again at the basic emotional responses and the different ways you can describe those states. I want you to consider what tends to dominate for you. When you feel under pressure, when you feel stressed, when you are thrown into something unexpectedly, which of these core emotional responses is your dominant go-to response? Just consider this for a few moments. This is an important piece of information to know about yourself.

Complex Emotions

When talking about emotions, we need to recognize that some of them are more straightforward, in the way they are produced, and some are more complex. But before we discuss complex emotions, I must emphasize the difference between not feeling and not expressing. We all experience emotions. Absolutely everybody does. But not everybody is connected to what they feel and certainly not everybody chooses to express what they feel. So when you meet people who try to appear as though they are cool about everything and they never get stressed or angry about anything, please know that is either a big fat lie or a complete lack of awareness on their part. Do not get fooled and do not ever think that you would like to be like those people who never get angry or fearful. Everybody gets scared, everybody gets angry, and everybody gets sad. It is normal. It is people who go out of their way not to express their emotions that I worry about. This means they are either disconnected from their emotions, which is bad, or they suppress them, which is equally bad.

Emotions are energy, as we already said. When that emotional charge is being experienced and it is not being expressed, it sits in the body and ends up imploding after a while. This is why somebody can have an intense emotional outburst, seemingly out of nowhere, with people around them having no idea where it came from. That emotion had been suppressed for a while and at some point, that bucket overflowed and the lid flew off. It is much healthier not only to be aware of what you are feeling but to express what you are feeling regularly. So give yourself permission to feel, be OK with whatever you are feeling and express it. It is the inability to express emotions that often ruins people's health. That is because that emotional energy has to go somewhere. Either we release it, or we will keep holding onto it until it builds up to a point where it will be either expressed abruptly (e.g., screaming, violence), or it will implode internally. In case of the latter, we will likely get cancer, an autoimmune disease, or some other diagnosis, or we will start to experience chronic pain.

We already know that the disconnect that many people have often comes from early trauma and is essentially an adaptation. Nonetheless, that adaptation can be quite damaging for our mental and physical health, as well as our relationships. We must also remember that this suppression or unwillingness to express emotions frequently comes from conditioning received in our early years, when you are being told that it is not OK to get angry, for example, because: *nice people don't get angry.* Or it is not OK to express love because that may be perceived (and often is) as vulnerability and weakness. There is fear behind that, of course. So if parents are scared to express their emotions, they will suppress it in their children as well. Often that is related to unresolved parental trauma.

So let us now look at complex emotions. Some emotions are easy to recognize, and when you feel them, it is pretty obvious that is what you are feeling. For example, furious. When people feel furious about something, they tend to be pretty clear that is what they are feeling. They may not want to admit it to themselves or others, but they can identify that feeling relatively easily. Similarly, something like a fear of spiders or other phobias are easy to identify. These responses happen without much cognitive processing. The same with being delighted or happy with something. You may go into detail of how that delight was produced; maybe it was because you felt comforted and it made you feel safe, or maybe you connected with something on an esthetic level. You can analyze it, but the point is that it is easy for somebody to identify they are delighted.

However, some emotions are more complex, and sometimes we may need to ask some clarifying questions to figure out what we are feeling. Those complex emotions are also called self-conscious emotions, in that you need to be a bit more conscious of self to identify them. They require self-reflection and self-evaluation. The emotions I am talking about here include: shame, guilt, pride, embarrassment, awkwardness, compassion, empathy, hope, envy, jealousy, remorse, boredom, contempt, awe, trust or distrust, and gratitude.

Let us look at embarrassment as an example. When a person is embarrassed, we are dealing with a set of behaviors unfolding over time. For example, a person may call somebody by the wrong name. Upon realizing that, they may gaze downward, suppress a smile, and shift their gaze. They may blush. There is distinct physiology associated with embarrassment. In emotions such as anger and fear, both heart rate and blood pressure increase sharply. In the case of embarrassment, research has shown that heart rate and blood pressure go up initially, but within a short period of time, heart rate slows down while blood pressure continues to rise. This may mean that embarrassment has its own unique set of physiological responses.

Most psychologists say that there is a significant difference between shame and embarrassment. I tend to agree with that. Some people intuitively think that embarrassment is just a weaker form of shame but that is not really true. Shame is a much more intense emotion, which is likely to be associated with moral transgressions, but most chronic shame is generated by people's unhealthy beliefs about themselves and tendencies to self-chastise. While people do feel shame in the company of others, "solitary" shame is extremely common. In fact, chronic shame is the most important issue to resolve, as it connects to identity and self-worth. On the other hand, embarrassment tends to stem from social slip-ups, and we rarely experience it outside of a social context. We do not tend to get embarrassed when we are on our own. Also, people who get embarrassed can often laugh it off. When people feel deep shame, there is no sense of humor associated with that feeling.

Now let us discuss the difference between shame and guilt. Although many people use words *guilt* and *shame* interchangeably, they actually refer to different experiences. Guilt and shame sometimes go hand in hand, in that the same action may give rise to feeling both shame and guilt, but they are not the same. Shame reflects how we feel about ourselves, whereas guilt involves an awareness that our actions have harmed or upset another person. In other words, shame relates to self and guilt relates to others. So if a person says or does something that harms or upsets somebody else, they might feel guilty about it afterwards. They might also feel ashamed about being the sort of person who would behave in this way. This distinction is important. We will come back to the difference between guilt and shame when doing work on self-worth and forgiveness.

What I also want to point out is that in order to feel guilty about the harm you may have caused to somebody else, you must recognize him or her as a distinct individual. So a person who struggles with separation and merger issues might not feel true guilt even if they were to use that word to describe what they are feeling. Also, many people who display narcissistic behavior often experience profound feelings of shame, but they do not tend to feel genuinely guilty because they do not have any authentic concern for other people. The lack of empathy associated with narcissistic personality disorder makes real guilt unlikely since guilt depends on the ability to identify and care how someone else might feel. In addition, when shame is so deep that it becomes somebody's dominant "trait," they usually feel so damaged that it is impossible for them to care about other people's feelings. Those people may view others as perfect or lucky and they may be envious of people they consider shame-free. All this is happening mostly at the subconscious level. This kind of shame is associated with severe attachment trauma, which causes psychological damage. The capacity to feel guilt is dependent on psychological growth, and that resulting psychological damage impedes growth.

Healthy Versus Unhealthy Guilt & Shame

Before we move on, I also want to emphasize the difference between healthy and unhealthy guilt and shame. There is, of course, such a thing as healthy guilt and shame. If you behave in a way that hurts somebody and you realize it, you feel guilty and you may also feel ashamed of yourself for behaving this way. Then you apologize and you get over it. You understand that you are a human being and you make mistakes. It is done. It was a normal response to feel guilt and shame in that instance. Then, the healthy thing to do, once you have issued an apology or performed some other corrective action, is to put it to bed.

However, these days people feel shame and guilt about anything and everything, and they feel it constantly. In my opinion, it is quite disgusting how society continuously shames us for everything: not being obedient citizens, not being good parents, not being hard-working enough, etc. Everywhere you turn, there is somebody trying to shame you and make you feel guilty for something. It is hideous. It is toxic. It damages people because it affects their core identity, and, of course, sooner or later it affects their health. A deep sense of shame can be, and often is, at the very core of somebody's illness. Recall when we were talking about secondary gain. It is very common for people to feel undeserving of good health. Or worse, they feel so much shame that they actually feel they deserve to be punished, and their illness is that punishment. They feel they deserve to suffer. So they do.

So this ridiculous chronic omnipresent shame and guilt that so many people have going on is, again, a product of early childhood trauma and negative conditioning (societal shaming). In addition, a person who got this core belief that they are not worthy will continue to reinforce that in their own mind and will attract more situations in which they feel ashamed and guilty. Plus, they will be more receptive to further programing by other people, media, politicians, and so on. Out of all the chronic emotions that people can hold onto, shame is probably the one that cuts deepest and is most toxic.

So as you can see, when dealing with complex emotions, we need even more awareness and more emotional maturity

206

than we do for those simple emotional responses. As I keep saying, we need to be able to feel in order to heal at the mental and physical level. Understanding emotions is also important because many people who do not have much emotional intelligence get really frightened with what they feel. That is because they do not understand what they feel or where it comes from. This perpetuates that constant activation of the fight-or-flight, and even freeze, response. As you already know, we cannot heal anything when we are in fight, flight, or freeze, so emotional intelligence is really important to healing.

Emotional Addiction

Believe it or not, you can get addicted to fear, anger, guilt, shame, etc. Biologically, when you have the same thoughts, behaviors, and responses, your cells adapt to the biochemistry associated with those responses. The cells will either modify their receptor sites to accommodate more chemicals that are associated with whatever repetitive response you may be having, or the cell gets desensitized to the chemicals since it is exposed to them repeatedly. So now you need more of those chemicals to have an effect. This means the emotion needs to be more intense now. Because of that your body will drive you to become angrier, more fearful, guilty, ashamed, etc., so the cells can get their fix. So your physiological need will now result in certain thoughts or behaviors to produce that more intense emotional response.

So you may pick up a fight with somebody and afterwards wonder what the heck that was all about. Or you may take more risks to scare the living daylights out of yourself. Or you may engage in a behavior that make you feel ashamed and disgusted with yourself and regret doing it shortly after. You then promise yourself you will never do it again, but then your body needs a fix again, and before you know it, you have "re-offended". And you run this pattern over and over, creating this downward spiral. Many people are addicted to creating doom and gloom scenarios, even when the reality does not warrant it. They cannot help themselves. That is because their physiology is now controlling their mind and they do not even have a clue that is what is happening.

Developing Emotional Intelligence

The first step to developing emotional intelligence is to become proficient at recognizing the core emotions when they show up. I highly encourage you to be curious when it comes to emotions. You know now that you do not have to be afraid of emotions because they are just energy in motion, meaning energy that is constantly moving. You now also have some tools to allow that energy to move through you. Remember, it is only when you resist this energy moving through you that you create emotional pain and suffering. Before we proceed with this work, I would like to make you aware that it is normal to sometimes have emotional detox symptoms when releasing emotional energy. I have included a video on how those might manifest and how to deal with them in the Additional Resources, so please familiarize yourself with that.

When you are not sure what you are feeling, you can ask yourself some questions. When you are emotionally stuck and want to ask these questions, I recommend that you close your eyes and make yourself comfortable. Take a few deep slow breaths and drop into the body first. Focus on slowing your breathing right down. The idea is to let the subconscious mind come to the forefront with a few minutes of relaxation because your subconscious does have the answers. Make sure that you put particular emphasis on relaxing the muscles around your eyes and relaxing the jaw.

When you are asking those questions, you must not over-think it but instead go with the first answer that comes to mind. Remember, the subconscious is faster than the conscious mind, so it answers first. When you start overthinking, you are attempting to get your answer from your conscious mind, but if your conscious mind had the answer in the first place, you would have already thought about it. By overthinking and overanalyzing, you are blocking your subconscious mind. This is, by the way, why people frequently have an instinct that they should act in a certain way but then they overthink it and let the conscious mind interfere. They act based on their conscious mind only to realize that the first instinctive response was the correct one and it would have served them better. I am sure you have had similar experiences before.

You can start with asking questions directly linked to the basic emotions, such as: *Am I afraid? Am I angry? Am I sad? Am I disgusted?* For instance, somebody can say: *I feel numb.* So what is that related to? Are you afraid? Are you angry? Are you sad? Are you disgusted? What is hiding behind "numb"? It is possible that what they are feeling might be deep sadness or fear or disgust, so it is worth asking these questions to uncover which basic emotion is being experienced. You may actually want to ask targeted questions: *What am I afraid of? What am I angry about? What or who am I disgusted with? What am I sad about?* If what you are feeling is really related to fear then by asking: *What am I afraid of?*, you will get an answer from your subconscious mind and that will tell you there is indeed an element of fear there. If you get nothing and that question does not resonate at all, then what you are experiencing might not be related to fear. Maybe it is disgust. So then ask: *What or who am I disgusted with?* and see what comes up.

Here are some other questions that may further help clarify what you are feeling in any given moment:

Is this feeling relating to myself or somebody else?

When did I start feeling this, and what where the circumstances?

What would happen if I didn't feel it?

How does what I am feeling fit into the big picture?

If I were to feel the opposite of what I am feeling right now, what would it be?

Cover-Ups & Distractions

We also need to recognize that some emotions arise in order to block our core emotions. I call them cover-up emotions. Shame, anxiety, and guilt are in this category. That happens either when our core emotions are in conflict with what we feel we need, with what pleases people, or when our core emotions become too intense and our brain wants to shut them down to protect us from the emotional overwhelm. We also have our distractions, which are used when we are prepared to do anything to avoid feeling our core or cover-up emotions. Common distractions in the Western culture include: joking, sarcasm, too much "screen time," criticizing, spacing out, procrastination, preoccupation, negative thinking, misguided aggression, working too much, over-exercising, over-eating, under-eating, self-harm, sex, obsession, depression, addiction, etc.

So somebody may be anxious about, for example, giving a presentation at work. As the time when they are supposed to do it approaches, they get some physiological manifestation of that anxiety; maybe they feel nausea, for example. Because they do not like this feeling, they might try to avoid it. They might start having negative thoughts, such as: *I can't do this* and/or they might start obsessing about something else unrelated that they "have to" do right away. So they moved from something that is essentially a fear of criticism and rejection, to anxiety (which is a cover-up for that fear), to distracting themselves from the real issue by doing something unrelated. This initial move from emotions to a distraction happens at the subconscious level and is largely automatic.

To resolve this constructively, you need self-awareness. You also need to be able to identify and connect with what you are feeling and use the tools you already have to help you deal with it. Once you notice your negative thoughts (*I can't do this!*), you are on the right track to get yourself out of this state. At this point, connect with your body and ask yourself: *what core emotions are driving me to have these thoughts and behaviors right now?* So in this example, when the person shifts their attention away from the distraction (negative thoughts that they cannot do the presentation) back to their body, they will be aware of feeling anxious, which as we said, is only a cover-up for their fear of criticism and rejection. Now they can deal with the feeling of fear by first acknowledging it, and then releasing the emotional energy using tools such as deep breathing, Havening Techniques®, or both.

If you are in a situation where it is not obvious what core emotion is driving your experience, you can use the questions I gave you in the last section to help you figure it out. If it is fear, you can ask yourself to make a choice. Are you choosing to fight, run away (fight-or-flight is what the overall purpose of fear is), or are you choosing to face it, given that what this particular fear is alerting you to is not a real threat to your survival?

There may, of course, be more than one core emotion behind what you are experiencing sometimes. In those cases, you attend to the emotions one by one. I also highly recommend that you examine what events and experiences in your life have led you to having this particular response in the first place and clear that. I will be teaching you how to do that later in the book.

Feeling Emotions in the Body

In order to become proficient in identifying emotions, you need to connect to where those emotions live in your body and what sensations they are associated with. I would like to now invite you to watch the video I have provided for you in the Additional Resources, in which I take you through exercises to connect with core emotions: anger, sadness, disgust, fear, happiness, and love. When you feel unpleasant emotions, part of what makes the experience worse is not being sure what you are feeling and why. By identifying what you are feeling, you immediately gain some distance and perspective from the feeling.

Be aware that when you are working with emotions, this is energy-consuming and it is normal to feel tired afterwards. If you experience that, simply take it easy for the rest of the day and you will be fine. Even though changing your neurology is an energy-demanding process, not dealing with stuck emotions is what drains your neural energy on an ongoing basis. When you successfully work through your emotional challenges, you can then start rebuilding your neural energy pool. If you develop greater control over your emotions, you will be emotionally healthier and more resilient and you will also enjoy more choices in your life. People who choose not to deal with their emotional hang-ups and triggers will always be drained by them.

Identifying & Addressing Emotional Triggers

Emotions do not just happen to you; they are a result of your nervous system being triggered to respond. Basically, an emotional response is a reaction to perceived events or perceived situations. Both emotional triggers and emotional reactions are personal and internal. They are not in the environment. Again, emotion means energy in motion. It is the label we attach to this movement of energy that determines its meaning. I would also like to reiterate: YOUR EMOTIONS ARE NOT CAUSING YOU PAIN. IT IS YOUR INABILITY TO LET GO OF YOUR EMOTIONS THAT IS HURTING YOU. It is all about resistance. I keep coming back to these golden rules of emotional work because without accepting them and applying them, you will not be able to master your emotions.

Think about being on a rollercoaster. You want to be that person who throws their arms up in the air, lets, go and has a great time, not the one who holds on to the security bar so tight their knuckles go white and wants to throw up afterwards. The more comfortable you become with feeling emotions, the less impactful they are. When you learn to identify and process emotions, certain emotional states actually become less intense. Why? Again, it is the resistance that makes them worse. Part of resistance is not wanting to feel something out of fear that it is going to be unpleasant and overwhelming. Your brain needs to get used to the idea that when an emotion comes up, you feel it, you let it be what it is, and you let it work through you. When it does, that eliminates the fear of having that emotion arise and being overwhelmed by it.

So let us look more closely at emotional triggers now. Identifying your triggers will help you massively when dealing with unwanted emotional states. It is because these triggers can be quickly changed, modified, and even removed! An emotional trigger is anything that sparks an intense emotional reaction, regardless of your current mood. This includes: memories, experiences, events, uncomfortable topics, another person's words or actions, and even your own behaviors.

Common situations that trigger intense emotions include: rejection, betrayal, being ignored or excluded, unjust treatment, being yelled at, being violated or having your boundaries violated, having your beliefs challenged, helplessness, loss of control or somebody trying to control you, somebody else's anger, lack of respect, disapproval, judgment or criticism, feeling unwanted or not needed, people being unavailable, feeling smothered or too needed, feeling insecure for whatever reason, somebody blaming or shaming you, perceived failure, loss of independence, loss of freedom, somebody's sexual advances, and unexpected changes of circumstances. This is not an exhaustive list, but these are some of the most common triggers. People can be triggered by one or more of these, and we all have different triggers depending on our history of trauma and emotional stress.

It is really helpful to first identify your triggers and then figure out why you have a given response. Perhaps, as an adult you get triggered by somebody ignoring you, and when you spend a moment thinking about it, you realize that your parents did not pay you much attention when you were child. Or maybe you get triggered whenever somebody is critical of you and you realize that is because one of your parents (or both) was extremely critical of you when you were a child. When you are looking at your triggers, it will almost always lead you back to your younger years, although there might be times when you are triggered by something as a result of a trauma that happened later in your life.

Let us take, for example, somebody being sexually assaulted. If they do not heal that trauma, they will very likely be repulsed or frightened by people making sexual advances towards them. They might respond with fear and/or aggression. In the case of triggers that go back to events from childhood, what we are dealing with is your inner child being wounded. When you as an adult are faced with a situation that remotely reminds you of what happened in your childhood, you will be triggered and your wounded inner child will come to the forefront, usually having an emotional response of fear, sadness, anger, or disgust.

Overcompensation

At this point I want to talk about overcompensation patterns that many people develop as a result of early trauma. For overcompensation to develop, a child must be pushed to their emotional limits in some way, but please remember that that those limits are defined internally by the child. It is about what the child is experiencing internally at that moment, and whether others think it's a big deal or not is irrelevant. A child can get traumatized by having the cutest puppy lick his or her face. When everybody around them just laughs and thinks this is the cutest thing they have ever seen, the child could be going through an internal horror.

Obviously, in this example, the child will probably scream or cry, and you would hope that the people around would get an idea that the child is not happy and would respond accordingly, but the point is that the internal experience of the child is 100 percent subjective and it is the only perspective that matters. So, when you are recalling your childhood, do not dismiss your early experiences. Do not just look at them from your adult perspective. You need to consider it from the point of view of your younger self and what you likely experienced at that time.

So let us look at some examples of overcompensatory behaviors. Often when people feel inferior, weak or lacking in some way in one area, they try to compensate for it in some way. So, overcompensation involves trying to make up for the feelings of inferiority by being driven to actual excellence or perceived excellence in either the same or another field. I want to emphasize how this works specifically when it comes to core emotions and what behaviors that tends to produce. The most obvious example is control. When a child feels out of control in whatever area, they will develop controlling behaviors in other areas. This is often the case when children are abused, or when there is a trauma such as death or illness in the family, or parental divorce. To most children these kinds of experiences are associated with complete loss of control. But again, this is about the subjective internal response of the child, so it does not matter what the event is as long as there is this extreme loss of control being experienced. The resulting behaviors can be OCD-type behaviors, wanting to be "perfect" at an activity, cleaning obsessively, eating disorders to control weight, obsessive exercising, etc.

What is linked closely to loss of control is failure. People who felt they failed a lot as children, or they were told they were failures, will most likely spend their adult lives overcompensating and always trying to get everything right. They will run away from failure like you would from a fire-spitting dragon. This may be as a result of repetitive scaring or a one-off incident that was particularly impactful. Type 1 on the Enneagram at its lowest expression is the most obvious example of this adaptation. Just to be clear, other Enneagram types can also develop this pattern. Interestingly, this overcompensation pattern does not always have to be destructive. Successful athletes, business people, and others have channeled their deepest fears and feelings of inadequacy into something positive.

Another example of overcompensation is a child who suffers neglect or abuse or is denied emotional nurturing, which results in developing self-loathing and quite possibly feeling emotionally numb. They might dissociate to a point when they do not feel anything and then in order to feel, they might overcompensate with self-harm or other destructive behaviors such as addictions. Another overcompensation pattern is when a child suffers a lot of rejection and becomes a complete doormat as an adult. They so desperately want acceptance to compensate for all those feelings of rejection that they let people walk all over them and take advantage. Often these people end up in toxic or even abusive relationships. The lowest expression of type 2 on the Enneagram is the most obvious example, but other types can also display this pattern.

Here is another example. If a child is mistreated, then as an adult they could respond with aggression in any situation that remotely resembles what they experienced in their early years. Often with people who are extremely aggressive and always respond with anger, there might be a history of abuse, but at the very least, there must have been some sort of violation of boundaries or lack of respect. And what about overcompensating for deep sadness with extreme joy? I am sure you have heard that many excellent comedians actually have a history of depression.

To understand developing and dealing with overcompensation patterns, think about a pendulum. In most cases, early trauma or early exposure to stress makes the pendulum swing to one extreme (e.g., extreme loss of control). What then tends to happen, as the brain tries to figure out how to survive, is that we swing to the other extreme. That is when we overcompensate. For example, that extreme loss of control results in being overly controlling in one or more areas of life. It is only when we become aware and do some self-development and trauma work that the pendulum returns to the middle and we become balanced. If we do not do this work, we are likely to swing back and forth between those extremes. This will cause us to experience those intense emotions that make us miserable and have the behaviors that can make our lives extremely difficult.

I have just mentioned that overcompensation patterns are not always destructive. This brings me to a very important point. When people come to me with emotional challenges and traumas, wanting to resolve them, I always ask them: *are you sure you really want to deal with this?* Sometimes, when I can see somebody being destroyed psychologically and physically, I do not have to ask. But emotions are not always that simple. Sometimes the same emotional challenge that is messing one part of your life can be the very thing that is allowing you to be successful in another part of your life. That is when that question is relevant because it essentially boils down to choosing what is more important. When we are working on values and beliefs, further in the book, we will look at this more closely. But for now I want to give you a couple of examples of when somebody may not want to deal with their emotional turmoil.

218

One would be when somebody for example has a very successful career as a comedian and they do not want to deal with their sadness because that is what drives them and inspires their creativity. If they take the sadness away, they may lose their edge and they may not want to lose that. So the question is: *what is more important?* Somebody who responds very aggressively to being disrespected or violated may not to want to deal with their anger if, for example, they have an ongoing court case that requires them to keep that fire alive in order to win. I frequently say to people who are in toxic or abusive relationships that if they deal with their pathological need for approval and acceptance, the relationship will not survive, unless the partner gets a grip and starts treating them with respect. But most likely, the person doing the work will leave. So that is another consideration.

Another example is athletes. It is, of course, possible that somebody puts themselves through extremely rigorous, relentless training day in day out, multiple times per day, despite exhaustion and pain, because they want to. However, it is obvious to me that most elite athletes have some form of overcompensation going on. Usually, it is to do with fear of failure. When they have to wake up at 4:00 a.m. on the sixth day in a row, feeling stiff and sore all over from training all week, it is that thought: *if you don't, you will fail* that gets them out of bed. That is what drives them and helps them achieve. You can often easily spot it in the way they speak and the words they use.

There is this cyclist who is a multiple winner of Tour de France and also of other grand tours. He is clearly one of these people whose dictionary does not include the word *failure*. At some point, he had a really bad bike accident in which he broke so many different bones in the body, and was in such a bad state, that he was told he was unlikely to go back to competitive cycling. It took him about a year, and he was back on the bike, and soon after, he was picked to race in one of the grand tours again. So how did he achieve this so quickly? He did it because the moment he was told it would not be possible for him, it triggered him to work very hard on his recovery. He was not going to fail. This is the sort of drive that, in my opinion, is facilitated by the stick and carrot situation that some people have going on in their psyches. In this case, his psychological hang-ups may have saved him from a lengthy rehabilitation and clearly saved his career!

So that is why it is worth considering what our emotional and behavioral patterns are, where they come from, and if we want to deal with them or not. In most cases, all we need to do is to rebalance ourselves so the pendulum does not swing back and forth, but there are those occasions when you might make a conscious choice to leave it be. It always should be a conscious choice. But like I said, most of the time, all you need to do is to aim for some sort of a happy medium. For example, if somebody gets super angry every time they feel they are disrespected, they do not necessarily want to remove their anger altogether. As we discussed earlier, anger helps us set boundaries, so if it is removed fully, this person might become a doormat that everybody walks all over. So in this case, they might just want to deal with the excess anger and build self-worth so they do not project their insecurities onto other people and jump to conclusions that somebody is disrespecting them when that is not the case in reality.

Another Way of Identifying Your Triggers

For you to understand this method, I need to first explain the idea of strategy. A strategy in this context is a sequence of internal representations (what you see, feel, hear, or say to yourself on the inside), which leads to a specific outcome. It is basically a pattern of processing that allows you to do things. It answers a question: *how does something create or produce something?* As we go forward, this will become more obvious. As humans, we have strategies for nearly everything, whether it is learning something, making decisions, processing emotions, or dealing with reality. There are some questions we can ask ourselves to help us figure out what our strategy is for running a particular emotional pattern, which will also help us figure out specific emotional triggers for this pattern we run. What you will find is that each time you run a particular pattern, the way in which you do it will be the same. That is your strategy for that specific pattern.

So let us say somebody gets angry. Here are some questions we are going to ask them:

1. *How do you know when to be angry?*

2. *When do you begin to feel angry?*

3. *What lets you know it is time to be angry?*

4. *How specifically do you do angry?* (describe in detail what happens when you get angry)

5. *How do you do "not angry"? How do you know there are alternatives to angry?*

6. *How do you decide to be angry? How do you select which alternative to take?* In other words, since there are

alternatives to *angry*, you could choose an alternative, but in that moment you choose *angry*. So how do you decide to choose that?

7. *How do you know you have achieved angry? How do you know when you get there?*

By the way, if you are getting triggered by these questions, take a moment to analyze what specifically about these questions is making you triggered.

Now, we will approach this from a slightly different angle, still using the example of *angry*. First, think of a time when you were really angry. Go there now. Next, considering that particular situation, what is the first thing that makes you realize you are about to get angry? Is it something you see, something you hear, or something you feel? Once you have identified that initial trigger, what is the next thing that causes you to produce *angry*? Again, is it what you see, feel, or hear? Or is it something you say to yourself? After that, what is the next thing that happens? Again, is it something you feel, hear, see, or say to yourself? Continue identifying all the steps that eventually take you to being really angry.

Let me now illustrate it with an example. I am going to use my strategy for doing *angry*. So first, what is the first thing that happens for me to get angry? I either see or hear somebody doing or saying something that I consider disrespectful. That is one of my triggers for doing *angry*. Then, the next thing that happens is I get the feeling in my stomach that is alerting me that whatever this person is doing or saying does not feel right. Next, I will say to myself: *They are out of line. I will not stand for it.* Next, I am aware of the feeling intensifying and turning into full-blown anger. Something important to be aware of when looking at your triggers is that sometimes certain responses can get caught on a loop.

So for me this can be the case here, whereby I might go between having a thought of how outraged I am and then having an even stronger emotional response. Then going back to the thought—maybe details of how this person behaved—and then again back to the feeling. The feeling is likely to get more and more intense if I go round the loop a few times. Next thing for me will be expressing that anger because I do not tend to keep things like that in. This strategy will run the same every time to produce this particular response to this particular trigger. Even when the trigger is different, which, in my case, could be that somebody is violating my boundary or they are harming another person or an animal, for example, the response to produce anger will run the same way for me. It will be obviously specific to each emotional response and each individual.

So, as you can see, there is a lot going on with all these internal responses to the external stimuli. The four main internal representations that you are going to have include seeing, feeling, hearing, and saying things to yourself. Your sense of taste and smell could also be involved if, for example, you feel disgusted with something physical. However, for emotional responses, it is mainly your visual, auditory, and kinesthetic senses, plus self-talk. So once we know our strategy for doing *angry*, *depressed*, *scared*, or whatever else, it is easier to interrupt the pattern and make sure we do not get caught on any loops.

Back to my example. I can do a number of things to stop the loop. I could reframe what I find disrespectful so I do not get triggered by silly things and silly people that essentially do not matter and are not worth my energy. What I can do once the original feeling in the stomach has shown itself and I become aware of it, and then I get a thought, is interrupt my pattern before I get on the loop. That will stop me from winding myself up even more. To be able to interrupt a pattern, you need to be quite self-aware, which takes a bit of practice.

You can interrupt a pattern with the SCC method I introduced you to earlier: Stop, Change state (physical movement, humming or singing, counting), Counter (with something positive). In the case of my example, I may want to counter with a thought that it is not worth it and that I choose to be the bigger person. Or, if the situation calls for it, I may choose to confront the person straight away, rather than stew in the anger. Or I can use Havening Techniques® to interrupt the pattern. I have introduced you to a few variations of Havening Techniques® already, and this is another great application of this method. As you get activated, you can use it in the moment to change your brain wave activity, you neurochemistry, and your physiology. This helps you process the emotion quickly and effectively.

By the way, you can also use this knowledge of strategies to help you achieve certain outcomes, like public speaking, for example, or overcoming dyslexia (yes, that is possible). You may have a specific strategy to load your dishwasher, clean your teeth, or whatever else. It basically applies to everything, good or bad. Out of approximately 60,000 thoughts that we have per day, many are arranged in specific sequences to help you produce different outcomes. Anything anybody does well, you can follow their strategy for doing it, and you can then install it into your own neurology so you become better at it.

To summarize this chapter, when you understand that emotions are energy and all you need to do is feel it and move through it, you will not create attachment and allow that emotional energy to build up anymore. It is important to note that this is often difficult to do when you are a child. That is why most people have some emotional build-up that is anchored in their childhood. But as an adult, and as you are engaging with the techniques I am sharing with you, you can learn to feel the energy of whatever emotion and allow it to move through you without getting stuck in it. Remember that you are not that emotion and you are not the traumas that caused you to have those emotional responses.

The issue comes when people live too much in their heads and refuse to feel because they find it too scary or painful. When people push emotions down and try to ignore them, this only causes problems down the line. Just because somebody represses their emotions does not mean they are not feeling them, or that they do not cause physiological and neurological chaos. They do. But when you shine a light on this dark emotional energy, you transmute that energy. When you face that emotion you did not want to connect with, that is exactly what you are doing, and it is nowhere near as big a deal as people make it out in their heads to be.

It is safe to feel an emotion. It is not going to harm you. It is just energy. It is not your identity. It does not control you unless you let it. I know it may feel like that sometimes, but your emotions do not control you, unless you create resistance to them by pushing them away or attaching narratives and stories to them. The trick is to move through and dissolve old emotional layers. Then, on an ongoing basis, when something happens that warrants, for example, an angry response, you get angry and you process it there and then. You feel it, you let it work through you, and you let it go. You do not push it deep down like before. You feel it in that moment and once you have, you choose to let it go so it does not sit there and cause damage to your emotional, mental, or physical body.

Action points:

1. Watch the video provided in the Additional Resources (https://www.dr-eva.com/shs-resources). It will take you through specific exercises to help you recognize and connect with your core emotions.

2. Use the questions provided in this chapter to help you identify your key emotional triggers and strategies you use for producing your dominant emotional states.

3. Start practicing interrupting your patterns with the tools described in this chapter.

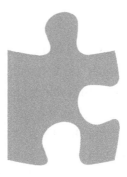

Healing Emotional Trauma

Encoding of Trauma & Its Impact on Health

Ann came to see me when her osteopath suggested her chronic back pain could be rooted in some sort of trauma. By this point, she had seen many different specialists and undergone numerous tests to rule out a range of problems. Nobody had managed to find anything wrong with her back, yet she was in so much discomfort that she was not able to get through the day, or indeed sleep, without pain killers. After almost two years of being on those pharmaceuticals, she was having many related issues, including gut problems, and she was very concerned she was now dependent on them.

When we started examining what could have possibly contributed to the onset of this problem, we did not identify any obvious events that had taken place. However, upon further questioning, it transpired that the day her back started being problematic she was out for a walk with her family.

There was nothing particularly unusual about the walk apart from the fact that they were walking past a viewing tower and decided to go up to look at the view. It was at that point that Ann's back started hurting. She thought she had probably overdone the walking and decided not go up the tower. When she returned home, she applied ice and rested, but the problem would not go away. After a couple of days of being in much discomfort, she went to see an osteopath. There was a slight improvement but not as much as she was expecting. A few weeks went past, and she was not really getting any better. So, she went from specialist to specialist, having many expensive tests. The problem became chronic, and nobody had any answers.

As she was telling me her story, I had a sense that not wanting to go up the viewing tower had something to do with all this. I started asking more questions to ascertain if there was a related incident in her past. Interestingly, Ann recalled a memory from her younger years in which she went up to a viewing platform on a school trip. She remembered a couple of her friends pretending they wanted to push her off the platform. They did not mean any harm—they were just being boisterous teenagers—but as they were trying to lift her over the railing and she was trying to escape them, she twisted her back, which she remembered being quite painful.

The whole situation did not last long, as the teacher started shouting at the boys to stop and step away from the railing. The teacher was very angry. She grabbed one of the boys, made him lean over the railing, and shouted: *Look down! If she had fallen, she would have died! You would have killed her!* Ann remembered that the teacher was very angry and shaken up, which made her realize that perhaps what they were doing was dangerous and that she could have fallen and died. She remembered feeling quite frightened and slightly nauseated in that moment. The discomfort in her back eased off fairly quickly after the incident, but the fear of what might have been stayed with her for a few days.

Ann had forgotten all about that situation until I started asking questions. However, when she started recalling the memory, she was still able to connect with the feeling of fear. We worked on this particular event using Havening Techniques®. Very quickly, she was no longer able to activate the fear. We then did some alternative memory work to neutralize her response to the teacher's reaction. All this was done in a single session. Her back started getting better after that session, and she was able to start weaning herself off her pain medication.

So because Ann's back was hurting as that emotionally heightened situation on a school trip was being encoded as trauma, that somatic component was connected to the experience. That is why the prospect of going up a viewing tower triggered Ann's back problem. Obviously, it is not always this straightforward, but this case study demonstrates the power of the mind-body connection and also how quickly trauma and associated physical issues can be resolved when the right connection is made and the right tools are being used.

Defining Trauma

Let me start by explaining a bit more about what trauma is and what determines if an event is traumatic or not. First of all, even though trauma is often discussed in relation to traumatic events and memories, trauma is not really an event. Trauma is a response. Even though events are important to document, and there must be an event for trauma to be encoded neurologically, this is not necessarily what causes trauma. Certain people can experience multiple adverse events and not be that affected. For some other people, an event does not even have to be that adverse, and yet they come away traumatized. So why is that?

For trauma to be encoded neurologically, a meaningful event must occur. In addition, the neurological landscape of the person must be permissive. This means there is a level of susceptibility to trauma, often because of a low level of neurological resilience. Finally, the person must have a perception of inescapability. Let us take a car accident as an example. In this case, there is an event (accident) and for most people this event will have meaning (*I could die*). If in addition this person's landscape is permissive, due to the body being flooded with stress hormones and maybe previous trauma, AND the person feels they cannot escape, this situation will be encoded as trauma. At the time of the event, there is fear present. The person will also likely feel loss of control and profound helplessness, as well as a broken connection to their body, to their sense of self, to others. They will likely feel ungrounded and experience a sense of isolation or loneliness. In the immediate aftermath of a traumatic event, it is common to experience shock or denial. A person may undergo a range of emotional reactions, such as fear, anger, guilt, or shame.

As we said before, if the person survives as a result of activating fight, flight, freeze, or complete shutdown, the same response will then be triggered every time the situation remotely resembles the original traumatic event. As I have explained previously, fight or flight, which is the sympathetic branch of the autonomic nervous system, activates first. If that fails to work, then the freeze response is activated. Muscles freeze. Breath may freeze at first too. If this continues, the body will go into complete shutdown mode, where heart rate and respiration rate drops, muscle become limp, metabolism shuts down, and endorphins are released so the person feels no pain. At this time, the person will not be aware of their surroundings anymore. This is an adaptive response when we cannot escape a traumatic situation. The trigger or triggers that will then activate this neural pathway over and over depends on how the brain filtered the external stimuli during the event. The key trigger for a person who was in an accident may be driving a car. However, they may be triggered by being in a car as a passenger, or even by seeing the same color car that they had this accident in. The brain may actually generalize to that extent.

We already know that most trauma originates in childhood, and that then makes us susceptible to subsequent trauma. We also know that unresolved trauma leads to the breakdown of the physical body sooner or later. I want to now have a closer look at the original Adverse Childhood Experiences (ACEs) study because that was the first major study that started linking unresolved trauma to poor health outcomes, and because of that it has become a landmark study. The ACEs study was conducted by the U.S. health maintenance organization Kaiser Permanente and the Centers for Disease Control and Prevention (CDC). Participants were recruited to the study between 1995 and 1997 and they have since been in long-term follow-up that assesses health outcomes. The study has very clearly demonstrated an association of adverse childhood experiences with health and social problems across the lifespan.

The researchers surveyed childhood trauma experiences of almost 17,500 patient volunteers. About half of these patients were female and the other half were male. Participants were asked about different types of ACEs that had been identified in earlier research literature. They included:

- physical, sexual or emotional abuse
- physical or emotional neglect
- exposure to domestic violence
- household substance abuse
- household mental illness
- parental separation or divorce
- incarcerated household member

It is very important to note the limitations of that study. As you can see from this list, there is no focus on emotional nurturing, or lack of it, which is the biggest contributor to developmental trauma. There is also no mention of intergenerational or ancestral trauma. When you completed my Emotional Toxicity Questionnaire, the second part of the questionnaire was focused on ACEs, so you already have an idea on where you are with that.

Despite the limited focus, the original ACE study found that:

- about two-thirds of individuals reported at least one ACE (in my opinion, this would definitely be higher if their focus had been broader)

- 87 percent of individuals who reported one ACE reported at least one additional ACE

- ACEs often occur together and have a dose-response relationship with many health problems (a person's cumulative ACEs score has a strong, graded relationship to numerous health, social, and behavioral problems throughout their lifespan)

- the number of ACEs is strongly associated with adulthood high-risk health behaviors, such as smoking, promiscuity, and alcohol and drug abuse

- the number of ACEs is strongly correlated with severe obesity and with ill-health, including depression, heart disease, cancer, chronic lung disease, and shortened lifespan

- compared to an ACE score of zero, having four ACEs is associated with a 700 percent increase in alcoholism and a 400 percent increase in emphysema

- an ACE score of six or more is associated with a 3,000 percent increase in attempted suicide and a reduced lifespan of 20 years

- eight or more ACEs triple the risk of lung cancer, hepatitis, chronic obstructive pulmonary disorder (COPD), ischemic heart disease and stroke, and increase the risk of chronic fatigue syndrome by 600 percent.

Those same researchers found in their more recent study from 2009, in which they surveyed 15,300 adults, that cumulative ACEs are highly correlated with adulthood autoimmunity. In fact, the correlation of autoimmunity onset in adulthood for women and ACEs is as strongly linked as smoking and lung cancer. They found that with two or more ACEs there was a 70 to 80 percent increased risk of developing type I diabetes, multiple sclerosis, Hashimoto's thyroiditis, Grave's disease, Crohn's disease, psoriasis, celiac disease, rheumatoid arthritis and chronic viral infections, lupus, allergic disease, atopic eczema, chronic sinusitis, inflammatory bowel disease, asthma, ulcerative colitis, and multiple chemical sensitivity.

So overall, they concluded that ACEs can alter the structural development of neural networks and the biochemistry of neuroendocrine systems. This means that unresolved ACEs can have long-term effects on the body, including speeding up the processes of disease and aging and compromising your immune system. ACEs contribute to allostatic load, which is defined as the adaptive processes that maintain homeostasis during times of toxic stress through the production of mediators, such as adrenaline, cortisol, and other chemical messengers. In other words, allostatic load is the wear and tear that results from the body and brain being under stress. Additionally, epigenetic transmission may occur due to stress during pregnancy or during interactions between mother and newborns. Maternal stress, depression, and exposure to partner violence have all been shown to have epigenetic effects on infants.

Other interesting research looked at brain changes that occur as a result of trauma. That research found that we actually get brain damage when we have those big one-off traumas. We have a shrinkage in our prefrontal cortex and, at the same time, we have an enlargement in the volume of our amygdala in the limbic system, associated with the flight-or-fight response. That had been previously observed in people with PTSD. However, what was also found was that people that were reporting chronic daily stress had the same exact brain changes and biochemical changes as people with PTSD. So if that perceived stress was chronic, that resulted in the same brain damage as those big traumas. So when we are talking about this perceived chronic stress, we are talking about feeling chronically overburdened, overwhelmed, being in a toxic relationship, perfectionism, etc. Recall all those symptoms of emotional toxicity we had preciously covered. What they found was that those chronic stressors negatively impact our brain in the same way that PTSD-type trauma does.

Before we move on, I do want to emphasize that all those potential negative effects can be neutralized by healing your traumas. The impact of ACEs on health occurs when the traumas remain UNRESOLVED. Even, if your health is currently suffering because of traumas, you can heal the body, or at the very least stop the traumas from further ruining your health, by resolving them! I personally had quite a few ticks on that ACEs part of the questionnaire years ago, but I healed my traumas and my biology, and I am enjoying vibrant health now, and so can you.

Tools for Dealing with Trauma

I have already mentioned briefly previously that in order to deal with trauma successfully, you need to use the right tools. You need to be able to rewire the neurology, reprogram the mind, heal the limbic system, and rebalance the energy field. Talk therapy on its own is never going to do it. It is quite an ineffective tool. This is why people who go to talk therapy, counselling, CBT, etc., which is not supported by tools that are able to achieve those deeper changes, go for months or years on end with limited or no results. They tend to know what the problem is and where it is coming from, sometimes they know everything about the problem, but they still have the problem. So what are some of the tools that are really up to the job? Some of the key therapies include: Havening Techniques®, hypnotherapy, Emotional Freedom Techniques, Somatic Experiencing, EMDR, NLP, and accelerated experiential dynamic psychotherapy. There are, of course, many others.

There are also tools like neurofeedback, but in my opinion, that is only going to work well if combined with belief change work and, of course, self-worth work.

I want to now talk a bit more about hypnosis and dispel some myths associated with it. This is because this is a very useful tool but there are some incorrect assumptions made about it. In addition, some people with certain religious views think hypnosis is bad. First of all, we all hypnotize ourselves all the time. EVERYBODY DOES. Hypnosis is nothing more than an altered state of consciousness associated with a certain brain wave activity. So if you are a human being, you self-hypnotize all the time. We spent most of our lives in a hypnotic state, actually. That is why it is so easy to program people. An example of that is when you watch a movie, which you know is not real and yet you have an emotional response as though it is. Same when you read a book. Daydreaming is a form of self-hypnosis. Also, when you recall a bad memory and have an emotional response as though that old memory is still your reality, you self-hypnotize. When we do guided meditations, it is simply self-hypnosis. It's funny that some people will say that hypnosis is not worth trying but a guided meditation is. It is the same thing! As is prayer.

This is why I find it quite strange that some religious leaders convince people hypnosis is a sin. It is essentially all about brain wave activity! The brain activity when people are deeply engrossed in prayer, sermon, or singing religious hymns is the same as when they meditate or daydream, and it is all self-hypnosis. If you are a living, breathing human, it is impossible for you not to enter hypnotic states! Moreover, if your brain could not access those states, you would not be able to function properly at either the psychological or physical level. Those are healing states. Obviously, when we do hypnotherapy, we use hypnosis to achieve therapeutic outcomes. I am utilizing hypnotherapy in my work all the time. Every time you do a visualization and you connect with it as though it is real, and create a physiological response to go with it, you self-hypnotize, like in the visualization we tried with the cakes.

One common myth, which comes from stage hypnosis, is that some people believe people can be hypnotized against their will. However, if you have been to a stage hypnosis show, you would have seen that they screen the audience first and they pick people who are the most suggestible to go on stage. Those people simply want to play along. Can they resist being hypnotized? Absolutely. 100 percent. If they decide that they do not want to bark or quack and make the audience laugh, they will not. But they want to have their five minutes on stage with Darren Brown, or whatever other stage hypnotist, so they go along with it.

In a therapeutic setting, as a practitioner, you must have people's trust. That is why the outcome of the therapy is 100 percent dependent on the quality of the client-therapist relationship and the resonance between them. I do not hypnotize the client; they self-hypnotize because they trust I can help them. **All hypnosis is really self-hypnosis.** The bottom line is that if I had a client in hypnosis and a fire broke out and I told them to stay in this state of hypnosis while I left the building to save myself, do you think they would just stay there and burn? Of course not. They would be out of hypnosis, running for safety. It would not matter in the slightest how much I wanted to convince them to stay in hypnosis and what suggestions they received. It is as simple as that. You are not unconscious in hypnosis (another myth), just like you are not unconscious when you meditate. It is an altered state of consciousness. That is all.

So what about hypnosis performed by the media and governments or mass hypnosis? Somebody could argue that people get hypnotized against their will and the programming still works. That is true, the programming works, but after all, people do choose to turn that TV on. They might just as well turn it off. This is a complex topic because the evil of this world that has infiltrated the media and governments knows how to program people. They are experts at that, and they use underhanded tactics, but you can still consciously reject it by not engaging with it, and there is nothing they can do about that.

Back in 2020, they performed mass hypnosis with COVID-1984. Why did it work so well? Because people kept engaging with the lies. Those who turned the TVs off early on were not as affected by the programming and were able to see things for what they really were. This was an example of trauma-based mind control. So in this case, people get hypnotized more easily because they have been plunged into fear and traumatized. Because of that trauma, and associated biological and neurological changes, they can then be programmed very easily. If you have heard of trauma-based mind control, then you know how nefarious and dark it is. This is really the only time somebody can be programmed against their will. Those other times, people simply let other people program them when they can just as easily be more conscious, say *no*, and reject it.

Post-Traumatic Growth

Post-traumatic growth is sometimes considered synonymous with resilience because becoming more resilient as a result of struggle with trauma can be an example of post-traumatic growth. However, in reality, post-traumatic growth is different from resilience. Resilience is an ability to bounce back after facing adversity. Post-traumatic growth, on the other hand, refers to what can happen when someone who has difficulty bouncing back experiences a traumatic event that challenges their core belief. They endure a psychological struggle, even something like PTSD, and then ultimately, they find a sense of personal growth through the process. It is a process that takes time and energy. Somebody who is already resilient when trauma occurs will not experience post-traumatic growth because a resilient person is not going to be rocked to their core by an event. They do not have to seek a new belief system. Less resilient people, on the other hand, may go through distress and confusion as they try to understand why this terrible thing happened to them and what it means for their worldview.

To evaluate whether and to what extent someone has experienced growth after a trauma, psychologists use a variety of self-reported scales. One of them, the post-traumatic growth inventory scale, looks for positive responses in five areas: appreciation of life, relationships with others, new possibilities in life, personal strength, and spiritual change. So, for example, people who had a brush with death, which made them question everything, will experience post-traumatic growth as this experience leads them to develop new appreciation for things that they had previously taken for granted. Post-traumatic growth makes you more resilient because when you survive a terrible trauma, you reinvent yourself and you grow from that. You then automatically become stronger and less fazed by life challenges.

Types of Trauma

Next, we are going to look at different types of trauma. We can classify trauma in a number of different ways, and I will present you with my take on it. The most obvious classification is to divide trauma from the point of view of whether the trauma was a result of a one-off event or repetitive events.

Event Frequency & Duration

Acute Trauma

This results from a single stressful or dangerous event.

Chronic Trauma

This results from repeated and prolonged exposure to highly stressful events (e.g., abuse, bullying, domestic violence).

Complex Trauma

This results from exposure to multiple traumatic events over a period of time.

Exposure

We can also look at trauma from the point of view of whether the exposure was direct or indirect.

Direct Trauma

A person suffers trauma as a result of direct exposure to an event or a series of events.

Indirect or Secondary Trauma (aka Vicarious Trauma)

This happens when a person develops trauma symptoms from close contact with someone who has experienced a traumatic event. Family members, mental health professionals, and others who care for those who have experienced a traumatic event are at risk of vicarious trauma. The symptoms often mirror those of PTSD. Secondary trauma might also occur if somebody witnesses a traumatic event occur to somebody else, as well as when people are repeatedly exposed to graphic details of traumatic events, for example, if they are a first responder to the scene of traumatic events. Believe it or not, some people can even get traumatized by watching a traumatic event, or events, on TV.

Other Types of Trauma

There are also other types of trauma that are important to recognize.

Pregnancy & Birth Trauma

This type of trauma is considerably underestimated, yet very common. This includes trauma as a result of any events or events experienced during pregnancy and/or birth by either the mother or the baby. I have already shared with you that this was one of the traumas I had to heal, and in my work, I often come across pregnancy and/or birth trauma. Unfortunately, in the Western world, people are still fairly unaware of how the emotional state of the mother during pregnancy and birth impacts the baby. This is compounded by the ridiculous over-medicalization of the birth process, which has got particularly bad since the 1980s. Women in the West have been programed that they have to birth their babies in hospitals lying on their backs, fighting gravity, and connected to hundred different machines and are led to believe that their baby wouldn't make it otherwise.

Many have swallowed this nonsense that their bodies are not capable of birthing safely without medical interventions. Thanks to this propaganda, there is an incredible amount of trauma that stems from birth. Why? Because a woman in a strange environment, away from what is familiar, connected to machines beeping all over the place, is not able to either run away or fight. She enters the freeze response. Of course, the baby reads that neurologically, hormonally, and energetically, and also activates this survival response. It is amazing to see that more and more women are learning about hypnobirthing and have home births. All the data we have in this area show clearly that home births, water births, and/or hypnobirths are the healthiest ways to birth if you want to ensure the best emotional start for the child.

Developmental (Attachment) Trauma

This is a very different type of trauma because as much as it can be a result of early childhood neglect, it can also result from lack of emotional nurturing. The consequence of that is the child not having their emotional needs met and inadequate bonding or even complete lack of bonding with their primary caregivers. As we already know from discussing attachment styles, our inability to attach securely stems from early childhood experiences. If we do not attach securely, we develop those different attachment adaptations. The brain develops from the bottom upward. Lower parts of the brain are responsible for functions dedicated to ensuring survival and responding to stress. Upper parts of the brain are responsible for executive functions, such as making sense of what you are experiencing, as well as gathering, structuring and evaluating the available information, exercising moral judgement and modulating your responses to the environment, etc.

Development of the upper parts depends upon prior development of the lower parts. When a child is not having their needs met, or is consistently neglected or abused, the stress response is activated over and over. This, in turn, leads to the sequential development of the brain being disturbed. The brain still develops, but because the proper foundation is missing, many things that follow are out of balance. Developmental trauma when associated with neglect or abuse can manifest in a variety of ways. Problems that can develop include: sensory processing disorder, ADHD, bipolar, personality disorders (especially borderline personality disorder), cognitive impairment, speech delay, learning disabilities, and more.

Most people with attachment trauma did not necessarily experience abuse and neglect. They just did not have their emotional needs met as children. Therefore, they will not necessarily have any obvious developmental or mental health issues later in life, but this type of trauma still affects their core identity, their self-worth, and how they view themselves and the world around them. This type of trauma is extremely prevalent, and pretty much everyone who has chronic health issues has this to heal at some level.

Post-traumatic Stress Disorder (PTSD)

This develops when the symptoms of trauma persist or get worse in the weeks and months after a stressful event (threat of death, violence, or serious injury). PTSD is distressing and interferes with a person's daily life and relationships. Most people who go through traumatic events may have temporary difficulties adjusting and coping, but with time and adequate self-care, they usually get better. If the symptoms get worse, however, last for months or even years, and interfere with day-to-day functioning, people usually get diagnosed with PTSD. Symptoms include severe anxiety, flashbacks, and persistent memories of the event. Another symptom of PTSD is avoidance behaviors. If a person tries to avoid thinking about the traumatic event, visiting the place where it occurred, or avoiding its triggers, it can be a sign of PTSD. There are many modalities that can successfully treat PTSD. Havening Techniques® is one of them.

Risk factors for developing PTSD include physical pain or injury, having little support after the trauma, dealing with other stressors at the same time (e.g., financial problems), and history of anxiety or depression. However, the absolute biggest risk factor for PTSD is childhood trauma. There is some research that looked at soldiers with PTSD and found that childhood trauma was a common factor. This is because of the impact of childhood trauma on the nervous system; it increases susceptibility to subsequent trauma. People with PTSD are often referred to talk therapy. As discussed previously, not only is this going to be ineffective in neurologically removing that trauma, for which amygdala depotentiation is needed, but it can actually re-traumatize people.

Collective Trauma

This is a traumatic psychological effect shared by a group of people of any size. It can include an entire society. Collective trauma not only brings distress and negative consequences to individuals, but it can also change the entire fabric of a community. Traumatic events witnessed by an entire society can stir up collective sentiment, often resulting in a shift in that society's culture and mass actions. Collective trauma can impact relationships and can alter policies and the way the society functions. It can change the society's social norms and even collapse entire systems. Some examples of collective trauma include wars, natural disasters, terrorist attacks, communist and fascist takeovers and regimes, holocaust, famine, recessions, the global pedophilia and human trafficking epidemic, and so on.

Intergenerational or Transgenerational Trauma (Also Historical Trauma, Cultural Trauma, & Social Trauma)

There may be times when your mind and body react to stories of trauma from your parents or grandparents. Trauma can be passed down generationally. Researchers shows that if an experience significantly impacts a person's life, it can be transmitted to their children, their children's children, and so on, until the cycle is broken. Your ancestors' fear or suffering can stay with you in ways that you may not expect. In case of historical trauma, we are talking about a complex and collective trauma experienced over time and across generations by a group of people who share an identity, affiliation, or circumstance (genocide, war, slavery, institutional oppression, and totalitarian regimes).

Cultural trauma is a related concept and occurs when members of a group feel they have been subjected to a traumatic event that negatively alters their collective psyche by forever marking their memories and changing their future identity. Cultural trauma forms three or more generations after the event. Because cultural trauma can only be recognized and studied retrospectively, it is prone to inaccuracies. Our memories are usually just partially true at best and often completely mythical.

It is worth noting that not every adversity becomes a cultural trauma. Adversities that result in trauma are often chronic and compounded. They tend to involve deliberate victimization and moral injury. Both historical and cultural trauma are imprints of collective victimization suffered by people, which obviously pose a threat to their mental health. Cultural identity is the driving force behind cultural trauma, and it reflects a collective sense of victimhood. Cultural trauma is also accompanied by a sense of trauma permanency, a sense that trauma has always been there (therefore, it defines part of culture) and will indefinitely continue into the future.

There are several ways that trauma can be passed on through generations. Researchers studying Holocaust survivors and their offspring were specifically interested in one region of a gene associated with the regulation of stress hormones. They thought that if there was a transmitted effect of trauma, it would be in a stress-related gene that influences the way we behave and cope with our environment. They found epigenetic tags on the very same part of this gene in both the Holocaust survivors and their children. The same correlation was not found in any of the control group or their children. Through further genetic analysis, they ruled out the possibility that the epigenetic changes were a result of trauma that the survivors' children had experienced themselves.

Furthermore, as we already know, experiencing trauma can lead to maladaptive ways of coping with unresolved emotions about the event. These coping mechanisms such as hyper-vigilance or avoidance may manifest as anger, anxiety, panic, depression, etc. This, in turn, will affect relationships. Because the human brain develops in direct response to the environment, the emotional responses of the parent will affect the developing brain of their child. Those neurochemical changes in the brain as a result of experiencing trauma can also be passed on. This is true for intergenerational trauma, such as slavery, genocide, war, and terrorism, but also individual trauma, such as rape, physical abuse, or extreme neglect. Both can have long-lasting effects over generations. People who live through these events, particularly collective traumas, often go untreated. Most are unaware that they carry that trauma or that they may pass it on to future generations.

In addition, a parent who has survived a horrific event might be in constant state of fear, anxiety, or depression, which will lead to a chronically dysregulated nervous system over time. This, in turn, can affect how the parent interacts with the child, leading to an insecure attachment style. This insecure attachment style then sets up the child to feel unsafe, insecure, and unable to trust the world. Through unconscious cues, such as the parent showing signs of fear or anxiety when confronted by "triggers," the child will absorb those emotions from the parent. Finally, trauma can be passed on by the message of a parent's storytelling.

Ancestral Trauma

These are traumas that occurred thousands of years ago yet remain embedded as genetic memories in the collective unconscious. Ancestral trauma can be experienced concurrently with personal issues rising to the surface for healing, or independently. We have talked about how trauma affects the nervous system and how it can get stuck in the body, but, of course, trauma can and does sit in our energy field as well. We can deal with ancestral trauma by doing ancestral clearing. This involves healing from inherited emotional issues, unhealthy patterns, or unresolved trauma from your ancestral lineage. When you do that, you release yourself from energetic patterns that are tied to your ancestors and can have a disruptive influence in your present life experience. Some of these unhealthy patterns can block your pathway to living your authentic life that you want to live and interfere with your sense of self or experiencing vitality and peace.

Ancestral clearing is based upon the belief that what happened in your ancestors' past is actually present and alive today within your cellular body and energy field. Consequently, your ancestors' unhealed emotional wounds, traumatic events, or damaging thought patterns or belief systems may still exist within your energetic grid. This grid connects you to the energy pattern of your entire family tree and it goes generations back. Most indigenous cultures, such as Aborigines and Native Americans, believe that their ancestors play an active part in their lives. For example, when making a significant decision for their family or community, they take into account the effects of that decision several generations back and several generations forward.

Remember that in the quantum field, time has no meaning in the way that it does for us on a conscious level. Past, present, and future are happening simultaneously. For that reason, when you heal yourself, you heal your ancestors and your descendants at the same time. Because energy is never lost but simply changes form, emotional issues or traumas that were not dealt with by your ancestors can hang about in your energy field, creating imbalances and blocks. Ancestral clearing can transform energetic patterns that are not in your highest good or are preventing you from carrying out your life's purpose.

Past-life Trauma

This relates to reincarnation and your past lives. If this is a step too far for you or clashes with your spiritual beliefs, that is OK. Leave this bit out and move on. I have to talk about it because this is something I have experienced, and I have had many clients for whom this was an essential part of their psycho-energetic healing. People often have behaviors, memories, flashbacks, dreams, etc., that cannot be explained by any other trauma they experienced, other than something from their previous incarnation. Most energy healers will confirm this. Many of them work with that every day, and to them it is normal and nothing unusual, but many people are not prepared to entertain the idea of past lives or openly talk about it.

To summarize, I want to emphasize that most people will have to heal more than one of these traumas. Meaning, their traumas will fall into more than one category. This is obviously particularly true for people with chronic health complaints. So hopefully, as you were reading, you were getting some ideas on where you need to put emphasis to shift yourself along on this journey. As we continue, we will first focus on healing those one-off traumatic events, as well as repetitive traumatic events. In the next chapter, we will look at addressing developmental trauma, and further on, we will look more closely at ancestral trauma.

At this point, I want to emphasize that I believe strongly that unless you have severe mental health issues, you can do most of your own work with the right tools and methodology. I have proven this over the years in my practice. This is what I mean when I advocate health sovereignty. However, if you have mental health issues, a mental health diagnosis of some kind, if you have PTSD or CPTSD, or if for whatever other reason you feel you need to be supported through this process, you should absolutely get support. Just remember what I said about talk therapy. If you are not sure what you should do, you can contact me via email for advice. Provide me with a brief explanation of your situation, and I will give you my opinion on the best course of action for you.

Identifying & Clearing Problematic Memories

Event Havening®

We have already used Havening Techniques® in a number of different ways. This time, I am sharing Event Havening® with you because with this technique you can essentially do much of your own trauma work with great and permanent results. We use Event Havening® to help us address specific disturbing or traumatic memories. Why do we want to do that? A number of reasons. Firstly, when people have unresolved traumatic events in their past, they will get triggered every time they think about that event (memory) or every time there is something happening that is even remotely similar to that past situation. That is because, as we already said, when we survive the original trauma (what we call a sensitizing event) as a result of the activation of the fight, flight, or freeze response, the brain and the rest of the nervous system is set up to respond the same way every time a situation resembles the original event.

Since we survived the first time, the brain sees it as a valid strategy to use again. This is regardless of how unpleasant an experience this is for us every time. It is also important to realize that the neurochemical cascade is the same whether you find yourself in a real situation that resembles that past event or whether you go over and over that old memory in your mind. However that pathway is triggered, it results in the amygdala activation, which further contributes to nervous system imbalance. In order to stop this old trauma from dysregulating our nervous system, we have to deactivate that neural pathway (depotentiate the amygdala), and we can do that very effectively and quickly with Event Havening®. I now invite you to watch my video training in the Additional Resources on how to use Event Havening®.

Identifying Problematic Memories

In this section, we are going to work on identifying possible problematic memories or events that need clearing and neutralizing from the point of view of emotional energy. Some of those problematic events you probably already know about because you may remember things that you found traumatic in your past. In this case, you can go ahead and clear them one by one using Event Havening®. Others, however, you may be uncertain about and yet when you analyze them, you will realize that they do indeed get in the way of your progress. It is important to recognize that many people do not have many, or any, memories from the first few years of their lives. Some recent research tells us that we can form memories in our early years but that the memories often fade over time. Young children's earliest memories tend to change over time and get replaced with "newer" earliest memories. Plus, as we already know, not having any conscious memories from childhood often has to do with trauma and dissociation.

We have different ways of dealing with implicit memories and explicit memories. Implicit memories are memories where we have no awareness or language regarding the memory. These are formed early in life, prior to the individual having language, but the body remembers what happened. Implicit memory systems store emotions, sensory experiences (sounds, smells, etc.), and assumptions based on prior experiences. Implicit memories cannot be recalled but they can be triggered. Explicit memories are memories associated with awareness and language. These memories are felt emotionally, and we are consciously aware of them.

Implicit Memories

These are things we remember at the subconscious level and do not even recognize as memories. For example, once you have learned to ride a bike, drive, or play an instrument, you do not have to remember everything you need to do in order to perform that activity. This is, of course, very useful. However, implicit memories can be problematic when they are triggered by something in the present moment that reminds our brain of a past traumatic event. In that moment, we become overwhelmed with an emotion. This can be fear, sadness, anger, shame, or any other emotion. Most of the time, in those situations, people who have not done any of this work will likely not be aware that they are being emotionally triggered by an earlier trauma and what events in the past those emotions connect to. In fact, sometimes even when you have done a lot of work on connecting the dots and piecing your timeline together, you still may not be able to know exactly where that emotion comes from.

Either way, when those emotions show up, as I am sure you know yourself, people often act on what they are feeling in that now moment, which might be completely disproportionate to the situation. For example, if as a child you were frequently criticized and it caused you to feel bad back then, in your adulthood, you may overreact anytime you receive criticism, even if it is constructive. Here's another example. You may be walking down the street and suddenly be overwhelmed with a feeling of fear or panic because you have caught a scent that reminds you of a dangerous situation from the past (such as abuse or mugging). Again, you may not have any conscious awareness of why you suddenly feel panicked, but your brain feels it has to protect you from that perceived threat, so it puts that neurochemical survival cascade in motion. Having those sorts of reactions can, of course, be highly disruptive to your personal and professional life.

So let's explore some strategies for how to deal with those memories. First of all, throughout this book, you are constantly presented with opportunities to connect the dots on your timeline. So if you have identified, for example, that you have fear of failure, fear of rejection, criticism, or whatever other responses dominate your life, I encourage you to consider what event or events in the past may have contributed to you being triggered and have those responses. Once you have connected the dots, you can build an understanding of why you have those patterns in the first place. You then continue to bring those connections to mind every time you get triggered as you reassure your brain that you are safe in your present moment.

I recommend that you use Event Havening® to deal with any memory or event associated with that undesirable response. If there is more than one memory, deal with one at a time, starting with the earliest one you can consciously remember. Even though, in the case of implicit memory, you will not be able to recall the original sensitizing event, you can heal any other times when you have had that response that you do remember, which will weaken that neural pathway. Often working with the earliest memory, or the worst memory, can make those other memories much less impactful or resolve them altogether. For example, let us say that somebody suffered abuse as a small child and as an adult they get triggered when being touched in a certain way. They do not remember the original event that caused them to have a fear response as an adult, but they do remember times in their past when certain form of touch caused them to feel fearful. We can use Event Havening® to work on those conscious memories and we can then use additional techniques to heal the inner child. We will focus on this in the next chapter.

Another example could be somebody who experienced food scarcity as a child and as an adult they hoard food and get frightened when they do not have access to food. In this case, this small child's needs were not being met repeatedly and they developed this adaptation strategy that says: *you must accumulate food so you never go hungry.* As an adult working on that issue, they can go back along their timeline and heal all those events when they remember feeling scared because they felt they did not have enough food. We would use Event Havening® to heal those individual events and then we would also heal the child who was dealing with this original trauma.

I have my own example of this. When I decided to deal with my abandonment issues, the original sensitizing event (the original trauma) went all the way back to the womb when my twin died while my mother was pregnant with us. Obviously, I did not consciously remember this, but time and time again in my childhood and adulthood, I experienced being triggered when I perceived I was being abandoned. I worked on those memories and I also worked on healing myself while still in the womb.

I have some questions for you that may be helpful when doing your detective work to establish what your emotional triggers may relate to. Think about a specific emotional response when you are asking yourself these questions. Some of those questions are inspired by Sandy Newbigging, so I want to give him credit for this inspiration. When answering the questions, remember not to overthink it. If you read a question and you get an immediate thought, that is the right answer. Even if it does not make much sense. Always trust your first answer and do not edit it.

Think about your problem now. This should be a specific emotional response that is not desirable.

1. What event (events) in your life is (are) the cause of this? What needs to be resolved for the problem to go away?

2. What age were you (if you know)? When do you think this problem started? What is the earliest memory you can remember?

3. What actually happened? Be associated to the memory (i.e. imagine being in your own body looking at the scene) and when you think of that time, what is the first person, place, event, or thing that comes to mind? Remember the earliest memory you can. Be open-minded to what might have happened at that time. Paint the picture of that problematic memory. Even though you may not be able to recall the original traumatic memory, use your imagination with regard to what may have been going on. If you are challenged by this task, think back to when in your life you did not have this problem and when you first noticed you had it? How long have you had it? And also, what was happening in the 12 to 18 months leading up to it?

As a side note, when considering your physical symptoms, you also need to ask yourself what had been happening 12 to 18 months before you started showing symptoms. Any small and big negative experiences during that time need to be healed. You also need to consider good things that had happened or got resolved 12 to 18 months prior to your symptoms showing, as the symptoms often do not emerge until the stress response is disengaged.

4. Why was it a problem for you then? How did it make you feel? If an undesirable emotion comes up and you feel badly triggered, haven on it while imagining the emotional energy leaving your body. Ask yourself what it was about. What happened that caused you to feel that way (the first thing that comes to mind)? For example: *I felt sad because I felt there was something wrong with me.* Or *I felt rejected because Mom shouted at me.*

5. What do you know now that if you had known then, you wouldn't have felt that way in the first place? Explore several possibilities. Find alternative ways to view the past in order to make it impossible for yourself to still perceive this situation as a problem. Neutral is enough. You do not need to be happy about it. Right here, you can employ a bit of Transactional Analysis. The bad feelings triggered back then are experienced by your Child ego state, but now approach it from your Adult ego state perspective and answer: *What do you know now that if you had known then, you would not have felt that way in the first place? I felt rejected because Mom shouted at me* is your Child self speaking. As you step into your Adult self, you might say: *She only did that because she*

had just got fired from her job and she was really upset about that. It had nothing to do with me.

6. For this to have not been a problem then, what would you have needed to believe? For example: *Mom would not yell unless she was really upset about something.*

7. If a friend had this problem, what advice would you give them to help them be more at peace with what happened? Assume that you know everything about their situation.

8. Now consider not having this problem in the future. How will you know you do not have this problem anymore? How does it feel not to have this problem anymore? What is that feeling, and where is it in your body? Close your eyes and take a few deeper breaths. Start havening and with your eyes closed and spend a few minutes visualizing yourself not having this problem anymore. Be in your own body. What are you seeing, hearing, and feeling? What are you saying to yourself?

These are just some of the strategies for making those implicit memory connections and making this more conscious so you can work with it. Sometimes, of course, that is not possible because, like we said, there may have been dissociation or because those very early memories faded away. If you get an emotional response that you aren't sure how to process, remember that you already have techniques for managing those situations, such as the Stop – Change state – Counter technique and Havening Techniques®. You can also visualize that emotional energy draining from your body and practice grounding yourself.

Sometimes, bodywork, such as massage and craniosacral therapy, also helps people release trauma that is stored in their tissues. Yoga, acupuncture, and acupressure can also be very helpful. Plus all the body-based exercises we covered in Chapter 3. If you want to go even deeper into these aspects of healing, particularly trauma work, I recommend you consider enrolling for my *Addressing Psychoenergetic Root Causes of Chronic Illness* online program, which is very extensive and is supported by me personally. One way or another, it is important to get to the root causes of those emotional triggers and ensure that we heal the origins of our traumas.

Explicit Memories

As we said, these are memories you remember consciously so you can use Event Havening® to address them right away. I highly recommend you draw a timeline of all the bigger and smaller events in your life. This is very useful and provides you with a map of what you need to heal. You can do it in whatever format you want. You can just write events in your diary, you can use a spreadsheet, a flowchart, or whatever else works for you. One thing I want to say is be careful not to dismiss anything. For example, it is very common for people to say they have appropriately dealt with somebody close to them dying when it is obvious to me that they have not. Grieving is a process that cannot be bypassed, and yet many people try to distract from feeling the grief because it is a painful thing to feel. It's understandable but not healthy for the nervous system and biofield.

You already know from learning about attachment styles that if you have an avoidant attachment style, you are more likely to dismiss your past and make light of it. You might try to convince yourself that your childhood was fine when, in reality, it was not, and the emotions have never been dealt with. This is because of this dissociation that takes place. Also, remember that just because you do not think something that happened to you as a child was a big deal from your current adult perspective does not mean it was not a big deal to you at the time. Often clients will say to me when recalling memories from their childhood: *That can't be significant, it is so trivial!* So I will repeat this again and again: your adult perspective is irrelevant. It is your younger self's perspective that counts. If something stands out for you, even if it seems trivial now, there is usually a reason why you remember this particular thing that happened, and it is often because it had a negative impact on you at a time.

The Order of Healing Trauma

First of all, there is no right or wrong order when dealing with traumatic events. When I work with clients, I will always go where the client's mind takes me and deal with what the mind is presenting me with. However, when working on yourself, it is actually a good idea to deal with all the one-off type events first if possible. This is because more often than not, you can deal with those events quickly, and then that is one less thing to burden you going forward. An example of this would be an accident, a parent leaving, or somebody dying. Then, you may want to tackle those repetitive traumas, such as bullying or abuse. These are quite impactful traumas that happened more than once, so you may need to work on all the memories available to you related to that trauma before it is healed. Sometimes you can collapse that trauma by working on the sensitizing event (when it first happened). When that first event is healed, it will cause a chain reaction in the neurology, and you might find that the subsequent events no longer have the same emotional hold as they once used to before when you have healed that first event.

Of course, as we said, you might not always be able to remember the first time something happened. In that case, go back as early as you can recall and work on that memory first. Then you might find that the subsequent memories are not as bad in terms of the emotional response they elicit, but you still want to do Event Havening® on them, following the timeline. If you have a difficulty recalling early memories, another thing you can do is to recall the worst ever time you were affected. As you haven on that, you will usually have other memories presenting themselves that were previously unavailable to you. If you have a difficulty recalling any memory because you may have blocked them, you can work on the emotion itself. This type of trauma work is more advanced, but I do coach on how to do this effectively in my *Addressing Psychoenergetic Root Causes of Chronic Illness* online program.

Watch out for Your Subconscious Mind Trying to Derail You

This chapter should function as an initial guide on how to approach working through those traumatic memories and events. If you trigger something you did not expect that feels intense, continue to haven through it. If it gets too much, change state, bring yourself firmly to your surroundings, and reassure yourself that **in this moment you are safe.** Remember that emotions are energy that is constantly moving. Let it pass through you, and it will. In those moments, your subconscious mind always tries to convince you that what you are experiencing is worse than it actually is. In the defense of your subconscious, this part of your mind does not know that what you are recalling is not actually real. If the memory triggers your fight-or-flight, which is what happens if you feel fear, anger, disgust, etc., it will try to get you away from "danger." The protective knee-jerk reaction of your subconscious mind is to stop you from accessing these memories and emotions, and once you have accessed them, it's to get you away from them. So you may want to reassure your subconscious that it is OK for you to go there before your start. Plus, remember, feeling safe in your surroundings when you are doing this work is paramount.

In addition, watch out for your subconscious mind trying to put you off or make excuses. Most comfort zones are pretty uncomfortable for people, but familiar problems mean safety. So you have to have this intention of wanting to step out of your emotional cage. It also means being willing to let go of your story. Your current narrative. As well as being willing to recognize that your perceptions are not absolute truths. I encourage you to be willing to go with it even though your mind will keep trying to divert you, telling you that you are not convinced, that you do not want to be doing this, that you have other things to do, etc. But, of course, be kind to yourself and if your mind is being evasive, always reassure it that you are safe. If you start getting frustrated and beating yourself up, you will make it worse, so please do not do that.

Finally, I just want to emphasize that if you are resisting something in your life right now, I recommend you put that under a microscope as something to be dissected, embraced, and dealt with. Maybe it goes without saying, but those very things you are trying to resist, push away, get away from, distract yourself from, ignore, pretend not to see, pretend aren't a big deal, etc., are there to point you towards what you need to shift in your life. The moment you start to recognize that you have resistance to certain things is your opportunity to shift into a better version of yourself.

So maybe you have an instinct that something is not right with your job, your relationship, or certain behaviors you may have, but you resist accepting that these do not feel right. You try to ignore those things, you try to make the best of them, or whatever. However, if you were to be honest with yourself, you know at a deeper level that something is not right. If you identify anything like that in your life, you need to scrutinize what is preventing you from accepting it, embracing it, and changing it. Ask yourself what you are fearing. When you identify what you are scared of, you may find that there may well be something that happened in your past that you need to clear in order to enable you to stop resisting and progress. Remember that whatever it is that is showing itself to you would not be showing itself (i.e., you would not be aware of it) if you did not have the capacity to work through it right now. Plus, resistance never goes away unless you embrace it, and for many people this is a fundamental block to making progress in life.

Action points:

1. Draw the timeline of your life with any events that stand out in your memory. This is a very useful exercise to identify what you need to work with, and as you do it, you will most likely trigger memories that you thought you had forgotten.

2. Start using Event Havening® on some of the events you have identified that need to be healed.

3. Continue using Future Outcome Havening® and Affirmational Havening®, adjusting when needed so your affirmations are relevant to what you are currently working on.

Attachment Trauma & Inner Family Work

Healing Your Wounded Infant & Toddler Self

Pete was one of these people who thought he had a pretty regular childhood. Nothing much to discuss. It was fine. Even though he had struggled with eczema and asthma as a child, he had not thought much of it until his skin condition returned in adulthood. Throughout his teenage and early adult years he distracted himself from his feelings with different sporting activities. It was only when he stopped moving constantly that his skin became problematic again and his unresolved childhood trauma started showing itself, asking to be acknowledged. As is usually the case, there were multiple layers to this physical problem, including biological, chemical, and dietary factors, but unresolved childhood trauma and associated energetic imbalances were absolutely a factor.

His parents did not mean any harm. They believed they were doing a good job. They simply did not understand Pete's needs as a child. That often happens when parents are emotionally detached themselves and are uncomfortable dealing with emotions. They expect their children not to express themselves emotionally because they do not know what to do with that. But just because the child is pushed into this left-brain dominant way of being does not mean the emotions they are repressing are not going to cause problems.

They certainly did in this case. Pete's frustration due to his repressed feelings and not feeling worthy of affection caused him to self-reject and resulted in an over-active immune system and inflammatory issues. It is not uncommon for children who crave healthy touch to have skin issues if they do not feel that need is fulfilled. In addition to the skin reacting when he was emotionally triggered, Pete had also developed some self-destructing patterns.

Whenever his deep shame and self-loathing as a result of feeling rejected and unloved were triggered, he would lash out against himself. His form of self-harm was to scratch his arms or legs so hard that they would often bleed. This then became a habit. He had no idea that this was all to do with his inner child feeling frustrated and unloved. At some point, he realized that he wasn't scratching due to his skin being itchy; he was scratching in response to what he was feeling internally. Scratching to "address" his feelings would then cause the histamine response and itching, which then caused him to scratch even more. Pete had repressed some of his emotions so much that it took some really deep work to encourage them to rise up again so they could be cleared.

The biggest surprise to Pete was that some of the memories he had, which he thought were trivial, turned out to be instrumental in connecting to his repressed feelings of anger, sadness, and shame. Even though as an adult, he did not think those past events were important in any way, they were clearly impactful for his younger self and therefore needed to be addressed. There were multiple layers to Pete's healing but the most important aspect for him was to heal deep shame and learn to love and accept himself. He needed to learn to be responsive to his own needs, rather than ignore them, and that it was OK for him to express what he needed. He also needed to learn to be more present in order to change some of the destructive responses that had become habitual. Pete's story emphasizes that you cannot dismiss what happened to you as a child just because you do not think it was significant from your adult perspective, and that you do not have to suffer abuse and neglect to have attachment trauma that impacts your physical health.

Consequences of Attachment Trauma

In this chapter, we are exploring attachment trauma. Ultimately, this work revolves around healing your wounded inner child. Why? Because that is fundamentally the worst consequence of attachment trauma: our inner child is wounded and needs healing. This is associated with feelings of not being OK, not being good enough, and not feeling worthy or lovable. Our identity becomes eroded when we have those beliefs, so we need to fix this because if our identity is shattered, nothing will be right in our lives. John Bradshaw, in my opinion, one of the greatest therapists who ever lived, who greatly influenced my work in this area, said: *The loss of your IAM-ness is spiritual bankruptcy.* This is very true, and it's why inner family work is the crux of my method. It is the deepest and the most important part of it. At this point, I would like to say that I am going to present some key information and strategies in this chapter. If you want to go deeper into this aspect of healing, again I would like to invite you to consider enrolling in my online program, where I cover a wider range of approaches and protocols to heal your inner family. This is very deep work, so it is good to have support while doing it.

I do want to emphasize that attachment trauma is very different from PTSD or a one-off traumatic event, and healing it requires a completely different approach. As we have already discussed previously, developmental trauma is often the result of seemingly invisible repetitive childhood experiences of being mistreated, abused, or ignored. These cumulative experiences could involve verbal abuse, neglect, or manipulation by a parent. But we have also said that this type of trauma is about the child simply not feeling safe, protected, and not having their emotional needs met, which means that often this is about things that did not happen, not just about things that did. Lack of consistent and reliable emotional nurturing can easily wound a child, so they do not have to be abused to develop attachment issues. We have also said that all this is about the internal emotional responses of a child and not about how others may view it.

Quite simply, in the first years of life, infants and toddlers need safe, predictable, accessible, and loving caregivers. In this environment the brain is able to develop in a healthy, normal sequence of growth. If they internally do not feel that is what they are getting, they will be traumatized, and their development might be negatively affected. This is how your inner child gets wounded.

When we are born, we have some spare brain capacity (extra cells) so that we can cope with a number of different scenarios. If our environment is safe and protective and our needs are consistently met, then those extra resources to prepare us for danger are not needed. We are less likely to be on red alert all the time and we develop secure attachment. We grow up trusting others and having a more positive outlook on life.

The reverse happens if a child does not feel safe for whatever reason in their environment. The neural networks related to secure attachment and social connection get pruned, and the ones that will have the child ready for danger come to the forefront. That defensive response becomes exaggerated, and trust is affected. That is the issue with attachment trauma. It negatively affects our trust in people and life, either by removing it completely or by making our trust blind. Either is bad news. Healing our sense of trust is key to restoring secure attachment.

Like I said, to heal our attachment trauma, we have to heal our inner family. What does that involve? It involves healing our wounded inner child and banishing our critical parent while bringing out our free child and our nurturing parent. If you do not heal your inner child, your wounded inner child will literally run your life.

Infant Stage

The four key developmental stages in your childhood are: infant (0 – 9 months), toddler (9 months – 3 years), pre-school (3 – 6 years), and school child (6 to about 13 years). Then we have the adolescence period from 13 years to mid-twenties. At all of these stages our needs are slightly different. Since we are all individuals, there are no absolutes when it comes to our development, but there certainly are some commonalities.

As infants, we need to be welcomed to the world, we need bonding, and we need to be nurtured. It is all about safety and getting our basic survival needs met. We are co-dependent at this stage and we are not conscious that we have a self. It is more about *we are* than *I am*. The way the bridge between us and the person we depend on is built will have an impact on our future relationships. At this stage, we feel about us what our primary caregiver feels about us. We need to be loved as we are, touched, respected, admired, valued, protected, and taken seriously. This is what is sometimes described as healthy narcissism. If those needs are met consistently enough, we will not have to try to compensate as adults for not having them met at this early stage.

When doing inner child work, it is useful to gather as much information about your family environment at that time as possible. If you already know bad things happened at that time, it is important to allow yourself to grieve and feel that. Certainly never dismiss any of it. If you do not know much about what was going on when you were born, that is OK. We are going to go through some questionnaires. There will be a questionnaire for each stage, and when you do them, you will get an idea about how problematic or how healthy each of those stages was and what effect it has on your inner child. When you go through the questionnaires, make sure that you connect to your body and feel for the answer. As usual, do not think too much about it. Your woundedness is a continuum, so the more *yes* answers you give, the more a given stage was problematic and is contributing to your inner child being wounded. If you get triggered, use Havening® and make note of what triggered you in your journal.

1. Do you have or have you had in the past an issue such as over-eating, overdrinking, or over-ingesting drugs or medications?

2. Do you have trouble trusting your ability to get your needs met? Do you believe you must find someone to meet them for you?

269

3. Do you find it hard to trust other people? Do you feel you must be in control at all times?

4. Do you fail to recognize body signals of physical need? For example, do you tend to eat when you are not hungry or be unaware how tired you are?

5. Do you neglect your physical needs, such good nutrition, exercise, adequate sleep, attending to your dental health, etc.?

6. Do you have deep fears of abandonment?

7. Do you feel, or have you ever felt, desperate or considered suicide because a love relationship ended (e.g., your partner has left you or filed for a divorce)?

8. Do you often feel that you do not truly fit in or belong anywhere? Do you feel that people do not really welcome you or want your presence?

9. In social situations, do you try to be invisible so that no one will notice you?

10. Do you try to be so helpful (even indispensable) in your love relationships that the other person (friend, lover, spouse, child, parent) cannot leave you?

11. Is oral sex the type of sex you most desire and fantasize about?

12. Do you have great needs to be touched and held? Do you tend to touch or hug others often without asking them?

13. Do you have a continual and obsessive need to be valued and esteemed?

14. Are you often biting and sarcastic to others?

15. Do you isolate yourself and stay alone a lot of the time? Do you often feel it is not worth trying to have a relationship?

16. Are you often gullible? Do you accept others' opinions or "swallow things whole" without thinking them through?

So, hopefully, you now have a better idea of how healthy or problematic your infant stage was. One of the things you can do straight away is to start satisfying your own needs that were not met very well then (or not at all). Start to pay more attention to your basic physical needs and bring in some corrective behaviors, such as recognizing when you are tired. Use things that comfort you and soothe you that have a physical element; for example, wrap yourself in a blanket, have a nice bath, or get a massage. When doing Affirmational Havening® focus on trust, having control, and safety. I also highly recommend that you write yourself a letter with your non-dominant hand. This makes it easier to connect to your inner child. If your infant self could write, what would they want to tell your adult self? It does not have to be long. Before you start, take a few deep breaths and tune in to that part of yourself, your infant self, then let the words flow. Finally, in the Additional Resources, you will find a Havening® video with a protocol for healing your younger self.

Toddler Stage

This period is called the separation stage. It is a counter-dependence stage, during which the child is starting to say: "No, let me do it." The child disobeys under the parents' watchful eyes. The child is still bonded but must oppose the parents in order to separate from them. This is called oppositional bonding, also called the second birth or psychological birth, and it marks the birth of the child's identity. The *we are* becomes *I am.* At this stage, children do not have emotional balance, and their behavior is often extreme—like little dictators. They throw temper tantrums when they do not get what they want. Parents need to set healthy limits, but if the limits are too drastic, that will damage the child. The parents need to model healthy expression of anger and good conflict resolution. Children need to know it is OK for them to express anger and that parents will still be there. If the child is not allowed to express their anger, they will likely have issues with anger. They will either repress it or they will overexpress it. Those issues with emotional expression will be then carried into their adulthood. Learning healthy conflict resolution is also essential for the establishment of intimacy.

As the child learns appropriate limits, they learn about healthy shame. As we have discussed previously, excessive shame is extremely damaging, but the child needs to learn those healthy limits to know they will not always get what they want. As we know, this is where our development often goes wrong, when we are shamed too much unnecessarily. We learn object constancy at this age. The child learns that Mom and Dad sometimes give them what they want, and other times they do not, but they are still the same people. The child learns that they might feel sad one day and happy the next, but they are still the same. If the child does not learn this, then as they grow up, they will be rigid and think in all-or-nothing terms about life. We also learn to set boundaries at this stage. That is why we say *that's mine* a lot.

If your needs were not met properly at this toddler stage, or if you were not allowed to learn or express things you needed to learn and express, your toddler self will be wounded. The possible consequences of that in adulthood include:

- deep sense of toxic shame and deepening of this spiritual wound - *It is not OK to be me. There is something wrong with me.* The wound can actually originate at this stage.
- people pleasing
- being highly critical of self and others
- addictive behaviors (if the child could not learn to say *no*)
- a sense of feeling isolated and alone
- issues with balance and boundaries, which can manifest in any area of life—either letting people take advantage or taking without limits with complete disregard for consequences if the discipline was not there at all.

The following questionnaire will help you work out how problematic your toddler stage was. Questions 1 – 9 cover the period of 9 – 18 months, which involves crawling, touching, tasting, and simply being curious and eager to explore the world. Questions 10 – 22 cover period the of 18 months to 3 years, which is the separation phase. Again, try to feel for the answer rather than overthink it.

1. Do you have trouble knowing what you want?

2. Are you afraid to explore new places or try out new experiences? If you do try them, do you always wait till someone else has tried first?

3. Do you have a fear of abandonment?

4. In difficult situations, do you want other people to tell you what to do?

5. If someone gives you a suggestion, do you feel you ought to follow it?

6. Do you have trouble actually being in your experience? For example, when you are on vacation sightseeing, are you worrying about the tour bus leaving without you?

7. Are you a big worrier?

8. Do you have trouble being spontaneous? For example, would you be embarrassed to sing in front of a group of people just because you were happy?

9. Do you find yourself in frequent conflicts with people in authority?

10. Do you often use words that center on defecation or urination—like asshole, shit, or piss? Or does your sense of humor focus on bathroom jokes?

11. Are you obsessed with men's or women's buttocks? Do you prefer to fantasize about or engage in anal sex more than any other kind?

12. Are you often accused of being stingy with money, love, emotions, or affection?

13. Do you tend to be obsessive about neatness and cleanliness?

14. Do you fear anger in other people or in yourself?

15. Will you do almost anything to avoid conflict?

16. Do you feel guilty when you say no to someone?

17. Do you avoid saying no directly, but often avoid doing what you have said you would by finding excuses or manipulating situations?

18. Do you sometimes "go berserk" and inappropriately let go of all control?

19. Are you often excessively critical of other people?

20. Do you act nice to people when you are with them and then gossip about and criticize them behind their back?

21. When you achieve success, do you have trouble enjoying or even believing in your accomplishments?

In order to heal your inner toddler, use the meditation and Havening® protocol I have shared in the Additional Resources. When doing Affirmational Havening®, continue to focus on trust, being in control, and safety but also on feeling worthy and accepting yourself. Different behaviors that will satisfy your inner toddler include: going to a market and touch and examine various items, going somewhere you have never been before and practicing presence, trying a new activity, doing some fingerpainting or attending a pottery workshop, playing in the sand, or making different noises just to see what they sound like. As before, I also encourage you to write a short letter from your toddler self to your adult self with your non-dominant hand. You could also express your toddler self through art, also using your non-dominant hand.

Healing Your Wounded Pre-School, School-Age & Adolescent Self

Before we move on to discussing the next stage of childhood development, I want to draw your attention to how the lessons we learn in childhood, and the strengths we develop, need to be strengthened in the later stages of our life. Essentially, those basic childhood needs and lessons get recycled as we go through life. During puberty, we begin the process of forming our adult identity and getting ready for leaving home (separation). At this point, we need to rely on trust we developed as infants: a trust that the world is safe enough for us to operate in. We must become autonomous. Our success depends on how well we did during our first counter-dependency stage in our toddler years. We can then use our social skills we acquired when we first started mixing with other kids to make new friends and so on.

Then again, when we create a family of our own, we start another cycle. Once again, we need to fall back on all the things we learned in the first few years, like trust, autonomy, boundary setting, emotional expression, etc. We even recycle these stages when we start new relationships and when we retire. It also happens with parenting. Parenting will trigger early developmental issues for people, and the unmet needs will come up again. Often this results in toxic parenting. This is why people coming from dysfunctional backgrounds will repeat the trauma cycle unless they heal their traumas. Traumas get repeated until somebody breaks the cycle. This is why when reflecting on your childhood, you need to look objectively at your parents' history of trauma and all the challenges they never dealt with.

When it comes to our relationship with our parents, we need to do the necessary work to ensure that nothing that our parents do or say, or do not do or say, can trigger us on an ongoing basis and put us in those chronically burdensome emotional states. Just to be clear, this is not about never having disagreements or arguments. You can disagree with anyone, and that includes your parents. If you get over it quickly, make up, and move on, that is normal. What I am talking about is your inner child being constantly fearful, sad, angry, ashamed, etc., because of what certain things your parents do or say. I encourage you to carefully consider this whether they are still around or not. Even if your parents have passed, various aspects of your relationship with them are still playing out in your subconscious. It is very common for people to get triggered by the memories of their parents doing or saying things long after they have died and not even be aware of it.

So that is one thing to consider. Another is to differentiate your conscious response to the question: *how do you feel about your Mom and your Dad?* from your subconscious response. Why is that important? It is because we can have a lot of incongruency around our parents and how we really feel about them. Your inner child wants to be loved and accepted by your parents. Your inner child's responses will be affected by trying to obtain parental love and acceptance, particularly if that was not there when you were a child. Remember, we need to consider this from your younger self's perspective. That desperate need for parental approval is one of the things we need to heal. On the other hand, if a child feels like the parents are a source of their struggles, he or she will want to reject the parents. Sometimes they even want to hate them. So this person can end up in a tug of war inside their head. They feel wounded and rejected by the parents, so they want to be upset with them or even hate them. At the same time, their inner child says: *But it is my Mommy and Daddy and I want them to love me and accept me.* This internal conflict is toxic to the mind and must be resolved and healed.

The problem is that even if you consciously think: *I am OK with what my parents were like and how they treated me,* if your inner child is angry or hurt, than those adult thoughts will not matter. Your wounded inner child dominates your subconscious and will dominate your life. It is easy enough to convince yourself that your relationship with your parents was fine, but if your subconscious mind does not agree, it will keep producing undesirable emotional responses and behaviors until your inner child is healed and no longer crying for parental approval and acceptance.

Pre-School Child

At about three years of age, we start to ask a lot of questions, particularly *why* questions. We want to know everything. We are trying to figure out who we are. We also start to form more beliefs about ourselves and the world around us. Hence all these *why* questions. At this stage, we are really egocentric. It is because we have to focus on ourselves to work all these things out. In addition, we also have to test reality to work out what is real and what is fantasy. We learn about cause and effect. Our parents are modeling relationships to us, as well as their individual roles, and this is when we imitate our parents' behavior more. We want to be like our Mommy or Daddy. We also imitate our heroes, sports people, astronauts, or whoever is appealing at the time and play make-believe and dress-up games.

There is much potential for creating toxic shame at this stage, particularly if the child does not "fit the mold" and cannot be easily categorized according to societal expectations and norms. I have worked with many clients with massive issues around sexuality, and it pretty much always leads us to this stage of their lives in some way. For example, children at this age are curious about their own bodies and when "caught" experimenting and playing with themselves by a parent, they usually get told that they should not do it. Same with homo-sexuality. Many gay people carry an enormous amount of deep shame, which again, when they want to heal, brings them to this stage.

They can obviously be affected by what happens during those other stages too, but this is the key stage because this is when children first start to become aware that they are somehow *different*. Both boys and girls are expected to display certain traits and behaviors and show certain interests. For example, boys may be expected to show more masculine characteris-tics and be interested in manly type activities. Likewise, girls are pigeon-holed and expected to play house and pretend to mother their dolls. When they do not do that, parents often feel uncomfortable and might even mock the child or express disapproval. That is damaging because the child feels that they cannot express themselves the way they want to; that they are not accepted. They feel there is something wrong with them.

The problems at this stage will stem predominantly from dysfunctionality within the family. If Mom and Dad are shame-based co-dependent adult children, it will be impossible for the child to learn what a healthy relationship should be like. Or what healthy intimacy is. When children have to fill the empti-ness in their parents' lives, this has devastating consequences for the child's identity. This is called vertical bonding, which is different from mother-daughter or father-son bonding. Vertical bonding creates a role confusion, whereby son or daughter inappropriately takes on the role of the opposite-sex parent and tries to play that role in the family system.

Essentially, the children can take it upon themselves to try to save their parents' relationship and therefore the family unit (enmeshment). This causes the child to feel confused and emotionally abandoned and has bad repercussions for their identity. The most common role distortions of this developmental stage are: the super-responsible one, over-achiever, rebel, underachiever, people pleaser, caretaker, and offender.

Let us now have a look at some questions that will help you work out how problematic this stage of your childhood was for you.

1. Do you have identity problems? Who are you? Does an answer come easily?

2. No matter what your sexual preference, do you feel like you are really a man? A woman? Do you overdramatize your sex (try to be macho or sexy)?

3. Even when you have sex in a legitimate context, do you feel guilty?

4. Do you have trouble identifying what you are feeling at any given moment?

5. Do you have communication problems with the people you are close to (spouse, children, boss, friends)?

6. Do you try to control your feelings most of the time?

7. Do you try to control the feelings of those around you?

8. Do you cry when you are angry?

9. Do you rage when you're scared or hurt?

10. Do you have trouble expressing your feelings?

11. Do you believe that you are responsible for other people's behavior or feelings? In other words, do you believe that you can make someone sad or angry?

12. Do you feel guilty for what has happened to your family members or feel responsible for your family members in any way?

13. Do you believe that if you just behave a certain way or mold your behavior, you can change another person or make them feel differently about you?

14. Do you often accept confusing messages and inconsistent communication without asking for clarification?

15. Do you act on guesses and unchecked assumptions, treating them as actual information?

16. Do you feel responsible for your parents' marital problems or divorce?

17. Do you strive for success so that your parents can feel good about themselves?

Again, have no judgment. Accept the result for what it is. Use the strategies I have shared preciously to start healing your pre-school self. This time I would like you to write two letters—one from your pre-school self to your adult self about your feelings, needs, wants, and concerns; the other from your pre-school child self to your parents. This second letter should have two separate paragraphs. One addressed to your mother and the other to your father. You should write both letters with your non-dominant hand. Let your wounded pre-school inner child tell your parents what you wanted and needed from them back then and never got. This is not about blame. This is about expression of loss. You may also want to express your pre-school self through drawing with your non-dominant hand.

School-Age & Adolescent Self

During the school age, the child builds on the earlier acquired strengths of trust, autonomy, hope, willpower, initiative, and purpose. They must now learn everything they can to prepare for adult life, including cooperation, interdependency, and a healthy sense of competition. There are academic skills as well, but they are far less important than loving and valuing yourself. If a child does not have a healthy sense of self, then their academic learning will be negatively affected. Children at this stage are quite egocentric and like to think that adults are wrong. They like to catch adults making mistakes.

Technically, children at this age should be happy and content, focused on making friends and curious to learn. However, in reality, the education system is often a source of spiritual wounding. The assumption is made that all 10 year olds, for example, have the same level of maturity. Your inner school-age child could have been wounded simply because you were in the wrong grade at the wrong time. Plus, the traditional education system is all about shaming and stress. It rewards conformity and memorization, rather than uniqueness and creative gifts. It encourages perfectionism, rather than striving to be the best you can be. Even if you are trying your hardest at a given subject, you can still be marked as average, or even below average. This will make you feel bad about yourself if you have actually given something your best effort.

Since we are all unique, which we are, we should not be constantly compared to others or somebody's dreamed-up ideals. That is not good for any child's psyche. When kids get *fail* marks at school, it is quite destructive to their sense of self-worth, particularly if the parents put a lot of emphasis on school performance. When kids fail and disappoint their parents, they can either become psychologically crushed and drop out, or they become obsessive, perfectionistic, and anxious when they do not perform so well. In addition to all that, teachers project their wounds onto their students—just like in dysfunctional families where parents project their wounds onto their children. In addition, at this age, if you do not fit in with the crowd, you can be picked on and bullied. The peer pressure and peer shaming at this time of children's lives is very challenging and can definitely be traumatic.

Here are some questions to assess the level of woundedness of your school-age inner child:

1. Do you often compare yourself to other people and find yourself inferior?

2. Do you wish you had more good friends of both sexes?

3. Do you frequently feel uncomfortable in social situations?

4. Do you feel uncomfortable being part of a group or most comfortable when you are alone?

5. Have you been told on multiple occasions that you are excessively competitive? Do you feel like you must win?

6. Do you have frequent conflicts with the people you work with or people in your family?

7. In negotiations, do you either give in completely or the opposite: insist on having things your own way?

8. Do you pride yourself on being strict and literal, following the letter of the law?

9. Do you procrastinate a lot?

10. Do you have trouble finishing things?

11. Do you believe you should know how to do things without instructions?

12. Are you anxious about making mistakes?

13. Do you experience humiliation if you are forced to look at your mistakes?

14. Do you frequently feel angry and critical of others?

15. Are you deficient in basic life skills (ability to read, ability to speak or write with good grammar, ability to do necessary math calculations)?

16. Do you spend lots of time obsessing or analyzing what someone has said to you?

17. Do you feel ugly and inferior? If yes, do you try to hide it with clothes, money, or make-up?

18. Do you lie to yourself and others a lot of the time?

19. Do you believe that no matter what you do, it is not good enough?

Adolescent Self

This is, in many ways, the stormiest time in our life cycle. Our healthy achievement of the critical tasks in this period depends on our strengths developed in childhood. We experience reformed identity during these years. Adolescence is a bit of a lonely and confused time because even if the person has many friends, they do not truly know who they are. They seek to have their identity affirmed by other people or achievements. They are not sure where they are going. They can now think in abstract terms, so the future, which is unknown, becomes a problem for them for the first time in their lives and a source of anxiety. There also tends to be a lot of awkwardness and self-consciousness related to the development of secondary sex characteristics and sexual feelings, which often feel embarrassing and strange. This is the time when that pendulum can swing to the other extreme for many. If somebody experienced shaming around sexual things, they can become very promiscuous. Children who experienced loss of control can become control freaks, and so on. That can, of course, start showing up earlier but will often reach its extreme during this time.

Here are some questions for the adolescent stage:

1. Do you have trouble with parental authority?

2. Are you confused about who you really are?

3. Do you think of yourself as disloyal?

4. Do you feel superior to others because your lifestyle is nonconformist?

5. Have you ever arrived at a faith position of your own?

6. Are you a dreamer, preferring to read romance novels and science fiction, rather than taking action in your life?

7. Has anyone ever told you to grow up?

8. Do you rigidly follow some type of guru or hero?

9. Do you talk a lot about the great things you are going to do but never really do them?

10. Do you believe that nobody has ever been through the things you have had to go through, or that nobody could really understand your unique pain?

Exploring Your Younger Self's History

Before are some additional considerations so that you can obtain more information about your younger self's history. This will further point you towards what may need healing. Some things you may want to explore include:

1. Who was around when you were a child? Where was your mother? Did she spend time with you? How much connection was there? Did she cuddle you? Where was your father? Did he spend time with you? Were your parents married?

2. Was there anyone with a physical or mental health problem or an addiction?

3. How did your parents discipline you? Did they use physical or emotional punishment?

4. Did you have any siblings? If so, how did they treat you?

5. Who was there for you? Who was there when you were scared or crying? Was there anyone who taught you the limits in a gentle way? Was there anyone who taught you how to express yourself in a healthy way? Who played, laughed, and had fun with you?

6. Were there any violations of your boundaries?

7. What can you deduce about the behavior of people around you given what you know about trauma, attachment

adaptations, etc.? What traumas were they likely to have suffered themselves in your opinion? You may not know for sure but maybe you just have a hunch that somebody close in your family was, for instance, sexually abused. Even if you are unable to verify that, trust your hunches. Assume these are true and see what understanding they can bring in about what was really going on at the time.

8. When you are considering your pre-school history, think about who was there for you. Who was your role model? Who taught you how to be a woman, a man? Who taught you about sexuality, intimacy, and relationships?

9. If you have not done so already, create a timeline of key events in your life from as early as you can remember, paying particular attention to what was happening in those younger years. Remember not to dismiss anything that may seem trivial to you now. If you remember it, there is a reason why. Not getting a valentine card or not being invited to a party may seem like nothing to your adult self, but if it was a big deal to your younger self, it needs to go on the list and it need to be healed.

10. Consider all the key figures in your life: parents, other family members, friends, teachers, pastors, etc. Then just spend a moment categorizing them into those who supported and nurtured you and those who may have wounded you in some way. You can then use this list when you work on forgiveness. It will also come handy when you express gratitude. You want to express gratitude to those who supported you. As much as it can be challenging, you also want to express gratitude towards those who have harmed you because

they have taught you valuable lessons in life. If you are not at that point yet, hopefully you will be soon.

To end this section, I want to emphasize once more that this work is a process and should not be rushed. I recommend that you commit 6-8 weeks during which you do the self-worth meditation I have offered in the Additional Resources daily. I also encourage you to: 1) do 5-10 minutes of Affirmational Havening° every day focused on safety, trust, and self-worth; 2) do Inner Child Havening°; 3) choose a few tasks to meet your inner child's needs from the list provided and do them regularly; 4) write a letter, as discussed, when your inner child gets triggered. Ultimately, you want to get to the point where you can say you love your inner child, you are very aware of his or her needs in each and every moment, and you fulfil those needs.

Forgiving Yourself & Others

Forgiveness is critical to what we are trying to achieve here, which is to promote a healthy mind, nervous system and biofield, and therefore, a healthy body. You cannot achieve that without forgiving people who have hurt you. It is also fundamental to forgive yourself. Otherwise, you will always battle emotional toxicity. You may have heard that forgiveness is for the forgiving. It is true. You are the beneficiary of the forgiveness work you are going to do. It is for you. It is not a cliché. It is a very important concept to take on board.

Forgiveness is not about letting people of the hook or making excuses for their behavior. Forgiveness does not mean reconciliation. You do not have to return to the same relationship or accept the same harmful behaviors from an offender. Forgiveness is about freeing yourself from being somebody's victim. You choose to let go of them so that they cannot pull your strings anymore and so that you are no longer, in emotional terms, at their mercy or at the mercy of what they did to you. Forgiveness is about healing the past and freeing mental energy for the present. It is not some sentimental or superficial process. Where real harm was done, this needs to be legitimized and validated.

It is important to have the right expectations, however. Forgiveness is not an on and off switch. It is a process. It is possible for somebody to just say: *I choose to release this and let it go*, use a visualization or another technique, and successfully forgive, but most of the time, forgiveness takes time. Remember again the difference between your conscious and subconscious position. The forgiveness process needs to be completed at the subconscious level, rather than just the conscious level. Otherwise, there is no alignment. If subconsciously you still feel victimized, then that will negatively impact your mind, nervous system, and physical health because you will still produce thoughts, emotions, and behaviors associated with being victimized. Forgiving at the subconscious level requires healing the inner child because in most cases it is the inner child who needs to forgive. You may also have to do additional work on specific traumatic events.

It is important to also distinguish between forgiving yourself and others. These are two distinct processes. You will always be victimized if you do not forgive all the people who have ever hurt you or upset you. So that is one part of it. You will also need to forgive yourself for anything you may have done that you are not proud of. This is about healing guilt but more importantly shame. When the harm was done by our parents, or people close to us, we need to acknowledge that. That way we take them off the pedestal we tend to put them on as children and we can see them for the wounded human beings they actually are. If we look at our past objectively, we will see that our parents were adult children acting out their traumas and limiting beliefs. Only then do we have the freedom to change the impact of our past.

So how do you know you have completed the forgiveness process?

1. You are no longer triggered by memories and people who have harmed you.

2. You have compassion towards yourself and others, as opposed to beat yourself up for what happened or things you have done.

3. You are able to express gratitude for the lessons you gained from those experiences.

When you work through forgiveness, it is a grieving process. You are essentially releasing anger and resentment, but you will go through sadness before you reach acceptance. You may already have a list of people you need to forgive. I will give you a technique to use to help you with this process shortly. You will find that in some cases, you may be right at the beginning of the grieving cycle (shock, denial, anger, bargaining, sadness/depression, acceptance, meaning). For example, when doing trauma work, maybe you suddenly remember something that happened to you, and your first response might be that of shock and denial, quickly followed by anger. In other cases, you may still feel anger at a person because of something they did, and you may even be stuck on anger. Or you may be stuck on sadness.

Often people cannot really bring themselves to feel anger towards their parents for what they may have done, but they will feel deep sadness. It is important to make sure that anger and resentment are not sitting underneath the sadness. This is very often the case, and when you start to process the sadness, your anger will come to the surface. You might not expect it because the anger has been repressed so you were unaware of it, but it is important to process it.

Eventually, we need to get to acceptance of what happened and what those people did, and finally create meaning. We still absolutely reject the behavior and call it for what it was, but we accept in the sense that we make peace with the past.

When we do this, it is very important to separate the person from the behavior. This goes back to what I said about the conflict we tend to have when it comes to our parents. On the one hand, we crave their approval (until we decide to cut the cord). On the other, if they have done us any harm or did not protect us, we will be angry, resentful, or frustrated with them. So one thing that you can do to deal with that conflict is to separate the person from the behavior. This means that you can reject the behavior of the parent. At the same time, you accept that fundamentally they are not rotten people and that the mistakes they made had been a result of their own traumas, poor self-worth, limiting beliefs, etc. This separation and understanding makes the forgiveness process easier.

As I said, we do need to accept that real harm was done and we need to own our feeling about being hurt, neglected, violated, etc. We then need to process those feelings using the techniques that I am giving you. Again, please do not dismiss this and watch for your conscious mind wanting to come in and convince you that you are absolutely fine with what your parents or other people did. You need to dissect it in the way that I am describing and be honest with yourself about how you are feeling about those people and what happened to you. If you have genuinely made peace with it already, then that is great. But keep in mind that you would not have emotional imbalances and triggers if you had dealt with it all. I cannot tell you how many times I have had clients who thought they had forgiven, only to discover that, that was not the case.

The easiest way to identify that forgiveness work is needed or is incomplete is when you have a disagreement with some-body about something small and this turns into a full-blown fight. Perhaps this is one of your parents or a sibling, and you start dragging things out from the past that they may have said or done. Or you are having a conversation with somebody who was not even in your life when you were young, and sud-denly, they end up triggering you, and you explode. They might be looking at you like you are from another planet because they don't have a clue what this is about. However, when you think about it, you realize that they said or did something that reminded you of your mother, father, or whoever. So watch out for those triggers. When people trigger you, you need to ask yourself what that is really all about. Tune in to the associated feelings and try to work out how that relates to your past. That will point you towards any forgiveness work you may still have to do. Finally, you know you have not completed the self-for-giveness process if you beat yourself up and are highly critical of yourself.

Forgiveness sets you free, like I said. Until you have forgiven, people will pull your strings and you will recycle the same feelings over and over. The unfinished business from the past will continue to contaminate your present. Also, unless you forgive, you stay energetically connected to your parents, like you have never left home. Forgiving means your child finally leaves home and can be truly independent. As an adult, it is really up to you to nurture your inner child. It is your responsibility. There is no point in waiting for your parents to change or apologize. You are waiting for something that most likely will never come, particularly if your parents are no longer in this realm. It is important to complete forgiveness work whether your parents are still alive or not.

When it comes to forgiving yourself, this can be even more challenging than forgiving others. This part of the forgiveness process is complex because it involves accepting yourself the way you are but also accepting that you are human and you have made mistakes and will make mistakes. You need to ask your inner child for forgiveness for treating him/her badly because when you are hard on yourself and beat yourself up, it is your critical parent lynching your inner child. Just imagine your critical parent self, whatever that looks like, a stern and mean person. Now imagine your critical parent beating your poor wounded inner child, scolding them, yelling at them, or criticizing them. How do you feel about this? Now have your nurturing parent enter this scene, pushing the critical parent away and telling them to get out. Then see your nurturing parent hug the child and make them feel safe. I encourage you to do this every time you are aware of your inner critical parent coming to the forefront.

If you have done things in the past you are not proud of, neutralize the emotional charge associated with those memories using Event Havening®. Remember to always conclude this with some affirmations or a positive visualization. It is also a good idea to analyze those situations from different angles. Consider what caused you to act the way you did, and you will probably find it is not black and white. You may also blame yourself for something that somebody did to you. This is common with traumas such as bullying or abuse. The person often blames themselves. As much as we want to take responsibility for our responses, it is important to call other people's behaviour for what it was.

A child who is abused, was not just "asking for it." Just because they were frightened to act or speak up does not mean the trauma was their fault. The abuser's behavior must be called out and rejected. One way of healing those kinds of traumas is to use Event Havening® on those memories and, at the end, bring your adult self into the memory to take care of your younger self. Have your adult self reassure them and tell them they are loved, safe, and protected. Then have your adult self leave them a resource that will help them feel safe and loved when your adult self is not there. You can also use the Havening® protocol I am sharing with you in the Additional Resources.

Other Approaches to Forgiveness Work

Below is another effective way to help you with your forgiveness work. I recommend that you use this method to work through the list of people you want to forgive, one at a time.

1. Take a few deeper breaths and drop into the body.

2. Start to haven.

3. Bring to mind the person you want to forgive. You need to be clear on what the problem is and what you are forgiving

them for. If there is no specific memory but more of a feeling or knowing that this person did something to you, then you can do this as your adult self. If you have a memory, be your younger self talking to the person who harmed you but bring your adult self to be by your side for moral support.

4. Imagine this person sitting in a chair opposite you. You can put a plexiglass wall in between you and them if that helps you feel 100 percent safe (you can hear everything perfectly through it).

5. First, ask them why they did what they did.

6. Immediately, in your mind's eye, switch places so you are now that person and you answer the question as them. So you start in your own body, sitting opposite your father or mother, for example. You ask the question and immediately switch and answer as the other person. Continue to haven.

7. Once you get the justification for what they did, you are back in your own body. Tell them how that made you feel. Ask them what they have to say about that. Switch places and answer as the other person. There may be anger, resentment, sadness, or other emotions coming up for you. Be mindful of that. Continue to haven.

8. Next, tell them that you reject their behavior. Tell them you condemn it, that it was despicable, or whatever else you want to say, and that you reject it. Feel what you feel the whole time. Remember, your adult self is there to protect you. You can say anything you want; whatever is weighing you down.

9. When you have said whatever you needed to say, be in your own body again and say: *I am choosing to start to forgive you now.*

10. Then see the energetic cords that connect you to this person. They connect to the front of your body but also your sides and back. Now grab a knife, scissors, a sword, or whatever you choose, and cut all the cords. Then see the cords burst into flames and burn down. Then imagine yourself and the person in two separate bubbles and see them drifting up and away in their bubble. Say: *I am releasing you now. I am releasing what you have done now. I am releasing the hold you had over me. I am freeing myself of that now.*

Another technique you can use is to write a letter to your inner child from your nurturing parent. Stepping into your nurturing parent, you want to apologize for not being there when they needed it and promise to do a better job from now on. You write this with your dominant hand. Then, with your non-dominant hand, write a paragraph as your inner child saying you forgive your nurturing parent.

Hopefully, you have connected with these approaches to forgiveness work. I really recommend that you take your time with this process and do this work thoroughly. Remember, it is not possible to have a well-balanced nervous system or true inner peace without it.

Attachment trauma = wounded inner child = erosion/loss of identity = unhappiness/destructive behaviors/illness

Even though you cannot change what actually happened, you can change your perceptions, meanings, beliefs, and roles you and others played and the tactics employed to cope. This will help you "rewrite" your history in a way and help you address your attachment challenges. When you have healed your inner family and completed the forgiveness process, you will feel more worthy and you will love and accept yourself the way you are, which will enhance every single area of your life. You will become more resilient. You will be able to live your life on your terms without projecting your insecurities onto others, without being concerned what others might think or say, and without being stifled by social convention. That is true sovereignty.

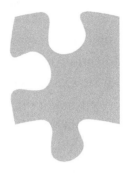

Values, Beliefs & Optimizing Your Programs

Prioritizing Values & Recognizing Value Conflicts

Christina's grandmother died at 66 years of age. She remembered her grandmother telling her about a dream in which she had a visitation from her deceased aunt, who predicted she would die at 66. Ever since that dream, Christina's grandmother believed she would die at that age. The dream scared her and at first, she tried to talk herself out of it, but in the end, she decided there was nothing she could do about it. She was a religious lady and concluded that if that was God's will, she would accept her fate.

Christina's grandmother did not really have any diagnosed health problems apart from elevated blood pressure, which was controlled by medication. Yet she passed away in her sleep a few weeks after her 66th birthday.

Christina's mother convinced herself that this was some sort of a family curse, and she too would die at 66. Despite people around her telling her that was crazy talk and it was not true, Christina's mother was stuck with this belief. She would often say things like: *We'd better get things in order. I only have X years to live.* Christina was angry at her mother for giving into this conviction and completely rejected the idea. She was horrified when her mother got cancer. Unfortunately, Christina's mother indeed passed away within a few months of receiving the diagnosis, "as scheduled", at 66 years of age.

Christina was determined that the *curse* would stop with her. She told herself not to be stupid and for the most part managed not to think about it for many years. But when she turned 64, the fear returned. She started asking herself: *What if this is true? What if this is going to happen to me as well?* She started having anxiety attacks and difficulty sleeping. Because she was not sleeping properly and she was a nervous wreck, her health started to spiral down. That is when she approached me. She wanted me to help her become healthier and combat her anxiety. She thought that way she could perhaps have a chance to avert the *curse.*

But in reality, this was not about having a healthier diet or lifestyle. This was not even about fixing the gut, correcting the sleep pattern, or becoming more resilient. More than anything it was about changing the belief that she would follow in her grandmother's and mother's footsteps and die at 66. It was not even originally her belief, but it became her belief as she witnessed what happened to her grandmother and her mother. Also, it did not matter how much she told herself not be silly or tried to distract herself or forget about it. The subconscious imprint was still very much there, and the fear it produced was debilitating. My opinion is that there was a good chance that belief would have killed her at 66. It was the belief that she needed to change. Having the healthiest diet and lifestyle in the world was not going to do that. Luckily, she changed her belief and she beat the *curse*.

In this chapter, we are taking a deeper dive into values and beliefs. The power of what we believe is immense and, as we have discussed previously, our values and beliefs 100 percent shape our reality. From the moment we are born, we are subjected to this social process in which authority figures, such as our parents, guardians, teachers, politicians, religious leaders, peers, and the media, define our cultural values, beliefs, ethical systems, and ultimately the way we perceive ourselves in the world. This becomes a problem if those perceptions are largely negative (which is frequently the case) and they cause us to experience emotions such as fear, anxiety, anger, shame, and guilt on a regular basis.

What Is the Difference between Values & Beliefs?

Values are quite simply stable, long-lasting beliefs relating to what is important to us. They become standards by which we live our lives and make our choices. A belief will develop into a value when our commitment to it grows and we see it as being important. Values are acquired predominantly through life experiences and other people's models of the world. Small children model their parents' and teachers' values. As teenagers, we may drop parental values in favor of peer values. We often pick parental values up again later in our lives, even less consciously than before. The adoption of other people's values in our early years is often at the root of inner conflict that most people have at some level. It is important to recognize that EVERYTHING you do is done in order to fulfil a value, even if you are not consciously aware of this.

How Do You Know if You Have Value Conflicts?

Whenever you feel anxious about making a decision or about having made a decision, this may indicate a conflict of values. In addition, using words such as: *should, ought to, must,* and *have to* indicates you are pressuring yourself to act on a value that deep inside you do not actually embrace. Whenever you catch yourself using these words, pay attention to the context. These phrases imply you would rather do something else, but you do not do it because you fear you may displease or upset somebody, or because there will be some sort of consequence if you do.

When you ignore or violate a value, you are likely to experience guilt or shame, or both. Guilt is a response to violating somebody else's value, and shame is a response to violating your own value. So when you feel conflicted, you need ask yourself: *What am I feeling?* Is it guilt, shame, or something else? You then consider the context and identify which value you have violated. One of the ways to neutralize feeling conflicted is to then find another value you hold which is important enough to you to outrank the value you violated. Let us look at an example of friendship versus freedom of speech. Many people have had this conflict recently. They want to be able to express themselves on social media or in conversations with people but because what they are saying does not support the mainstream narrative and the mainstream version of reality, they get "canceled."

They now have to decide what is more important to them: freedom of expression, and their own integrity, or friendship

301

with people who are not allowing them to ask questions or have a different opinion. If they value having "friends" who are prepared to ditch them just because they have a different opinion more than freedom of expression and integrity, they might choose to agree to keep the "friendship." In this case, they will probably feel shame for compromising their integrity. On the other hand, if their higher value is their right to free expression and their integrity, they will let this "friendship" go. They may initially feel some guilt, especially if they have known the person for a long time. However, if they remind themselves what really matters to them, they will soon diffuse that guilt and they will feel good about staying true to themselves.

The bottom line is that if we live our lives according to somebody else's values and beliefs that do not align with our own, we are not congruent and we experience emotional conflict. For example: *My parents taught me that I have to work hard and make lots of money if I want to matter in society, but actually what I value more is spending time with my family and friends.* In this example, if the person spends time with their loved ones, they are aligned with their own value. However, fear will soon kick in because, according to the parental conditioning, which became their subconscious program, their life can ONLY be worthwhile if they work hard and make money.

If they then decide to compromise spending time with their friends and family in order to work more and make money, they are violating their own value. To resolve this, they have to deal with the limiting belief they got from the parents: *I have to work hard and make lots of money if I want to matter in society.* They may also want to focus on another value they hold that is more important to them, for example, happiness. However, dealing with that limiting belief will be critical to their success in resolving that conflict once and for all. Remember that value conflicts are one of the main sources of emotional toxicity.

ANY ON-GOING EMOTIONAL CONFLICT = CHRONIC STRESS

Value Elicitation & Hierarchy Exercise

This exercise will help you identify what your top values are and what matters to you the most in your life. Once you know that, you can adjust your behaviors, activities, how you deal with people, etc., in order to be more aligned with your own values and avoid value conflicts.

Identifying What Is Important

List 10 things that are the most important to you in life (e.g., health, family, success, freedom, happiness, security/stability, integrity, authenticity, achievement, autonomy, balance, compassion, community, contribution, friendships, fun, inner harmony, knowledge, reputation, spirituality, personal responsibility, etc.).

Ask yourself the following questions to make sure you are clear on your values:

1. *What qualities would I expect to see in the best version of myself?*

2. *How do I interact with people, and how do I treat them?*

3. *How do I respond in a crisis or other difficult situation?*

4. *What qualities in my parents, grandparents, or ancestors do I admire?*

5. *What choices have I made in the past that made me proud?*

6. *What makes me angry or frustrated?* This could reveal repressed values you may have.

7. *What gives me a sense of fulfillment and meaning?*

Once you start to narrow it down, ask yourself these clarifying questions about the values you have identified:

1. *What is important to me about ?* (e.g., being healthy)

2. *How do I know when I am ?* (e.g., successful)

3. *What causes me to feel ?* (e.g., secure)

4. *What do I look for in a friend, partner, mentor or teacher?*

Ranking Your Values

Of the 10 values you have identified, which is the most important to you? Rank them now from 10 to 1.

Then ask yourself the following questions:

1. *If I had (your highest value), what would be the next most important thing to me?*

2. *Assuming I have* (list of values already chosen), *is* (value A) *or* (value B) *more important to me?*

3. *Assuming I have* (list of values already chosen), *if I couldn't have* (value C) *but I could have* (value D), *would that be OK?*

Now rewrite your list of values according to their actual importance, from 10 to 1.

Checking for Abstraction

What you find is that some of your values are quite big abstract values, for example, *freedom* or *happiness*. Some others are less abstract and can be defined more easily, for example, *being a good parent*. So now check that your number-one value is the most abstract and that the other values are contained within the higher value. For example, *happiness* is more abstract than *being good at your job* or *being a good parent*. If *being good at your job* or *being a good parent* makes you happy, then that is indeed a subset of *happiness* (alongside other things that make you happy). Now starting with the lowest value on the list, check if this value supports the actualization of the next higher value. For example, for some people, *having money* supports the actualization of *success*, which supports the actualization of *happiness*.

Motivation Direction

Now it is time to determine the underlying motivation of your values. Is it *away-from* or *toward* motivation? For example, if your value is *being yourself* because you *don't want to be fake*, you are stating what you do not want. This is *away-from* motivation. But if it is because you *want to be true to yourself*, then the emphasis is on what you do want, which is what we call *toward* motivation. Another example is, if your value is *honesty*, this may be driven by the fact that you *hate liars* or by the fact that you *respect and value integrity*. There will normally be one factor that dominates.

Why is this important? This is important because *toward* motivation is much more powerful than *away-from* motivation. To achieve anything, you need to have some motivation to do it. But here is a problem: most people do things because they run away from consequences of not doing those things, not because they truly want to do them. Of course, it is better to have some motivation than have no motivation; for example, *I eat vegetables because I don't want to be sick* is still better than not eating vegetables at all. However, it is far easier to maintain healthy habits when you do things because you want to and choose to; for example, *I eat vegetables because I like the way I feel when I do.*

Away-from motivation is hard work. It is fear-based. The only reason you are doing whatever you are doing is because you are scared of what happens when you do not do it. When you do something from a place of choice, it comes from a place of love, which is a much higher frequency. I am sure you already realize that it is easy to do these things you simply want to do. So when you reframe your reasons behind what is important to you, you change the focus and you change how your subconscious mind perceives it. That in itself goes a long way towards diffusing internal conflicts. I must emphasize though that there will be deeply seated underlying reasons why you are fear-driven, and this has to do with trauma and negative beliefs. When you work through these, you will start to discover that you are able to do things simply because you choose to and want to, not because you have to or should.

Clearing Away-from Motivations

Go through your value list and rephrase your underlying motivation each time you identify it as an *away-from* motivation, like in the examples above. If you do not do that, you can end up in a bit of a catch 22. For example, *making money* if driven by *not wanting to be poor* represents *away-from* motivation; running away from poverty, for example. However, the further away this person gets from being poor by making more money, the less of a motivator poverty is for them.

Checking for Conflicts

You need to check your values for any potential conflicts. Please refer to example I gave earlier on. This is because if you feel conflicted, not only will you experience emotional turmoil (chronic stress) but you will struggle achieving any goals that are connected to those conflicts. If you identify that you have a conflict of values, you will need to prioritize what is more important. This may require going deeper into why those things are important to you and it will probably mean there is some belief change work to do, which we are going to do next. You may also need to work on acceptance that you cannot have both. Knowing your personality traits and attachment style is very useful because it gives you a deeper understanding of why you hold certain values. You also need to double check that these are YOUR values and you have not simply inherited them from somebody else.

Living in harmony with your core values means you are living authentically without confusion, guilt, or shame. Just keep in mind that your values do change. You probably are aware that what was important to you ten years ago may not be that important to you now. This is shaped by our life experiences, as well as learning and knowledge we acquire as we go through life. So you do have to revisit this from time to time, making sure you are still aligned with your core values.

Identifying & Categorizing Limiting Beliefs

If you have been using Affirmational Havening®, you have already started working on remodeling your belief system, but in this chapter, I want to help you identify your key limiting beliefs and share some other techniques to help you change them. The objective is to assist you in reshaping your beliefs so that you can achieve your goals and have a happy life. Our beliefs influence all aspects of our life, including health. In fact, they make or break our health. We live our lives and form behaviors based on our beliefs. They even affect our DNA. Our body cells respond to our beliefs, which are essentially messages from the subconscious mind. The beliefs are then reflected in our physiology. Remember that an average person operates from their subconscious programs 90 to 95 percent of the time. In other words, we are physically a mirror of what we believe, just like, on the whole, our life is a reflection of what we believe.

Just as a reminder, our brain wave activity pattern from the time we are in the womb until about five to eight years of age is the same that you experience in a meditative state. Alpha and theta brain wave dominance causes us to be particularly open to hypnotic suggestion at that time. This means during that timeframe of development, we easily absorb ideas into our psyche. We also take things at face value. That is when we develop our foundational belief systems, and it just so happens that we are extremely suggestible at that stage of our life. The majority of the suggestions we absorb into our psyche come from our parents, other adults in our lives, school, society, television, radio, religion, and culture in general. We also build our belief systems based on our direct experience of the external and as a result of inheriting programs from our ancestors.

How the world responds to us is an indicator of our beliefs about our worthiness, whether we are loved, accepted, valued, etc. When we feel unworthy or believe people will always hurt us, abandon us, or whatever else, we see the world through these lenses, and we will definitely find what we are looking for.

What you believe, you expect, and what you expect becomes your reality. If you believe the world is unsafe, you will be blind to everything that gives you safety and you will see danger everywhere. If you believe that people cannot be trusted and they only take advantage of you, it is because of this belief that you will attract people who take advantage of you, therefore confirming your original hypothesis (belief).

If you are not sure what limiting beliefs you have that you need to change, look at your life. What are you unhappy with? What is not working for you? What are the worst things in your life? Where do you feel most limited? Again, from the moment we are born, we are programed with other people's beliefs of how life is and how we should live it. Most beliefs have little to do with reality, yet people live by them as their absolute truths. If you want to free yourself from those limitations that have been put on you by others and yourself, at some point, you need to step out of the matrix and FEEL for your own truths. Feel for what resonates. The moment you shift your beliefs and empower yourself, your whole world changes for the better because the frequencies you are putting out change and because you are now looking for confirmations of beliefs that are positive.

When you are too attached to your beliefs or you have made your beliefs part of your identity, it is more challenging to shift them. Keep in mind that when Copernicus first said it was the Earth that revolved around the sun, not the other way round, people were appalled. They had a different belief, and many struggled to entertain that the reality could be different to what they had believed. So be careful not to attach to your beliefs because we live in times when many common beliefs people hold are being and will continue to be crushed. If you remain closed and attached, you will struggle with this process of evolution that humanity is going through. On the other hand, if you remain open and accept that you are not your beliefs, and that there are alternative truths out there to the ones you have been programed with, you will have an easier time navigating through this. Relax and feel what resonates. Have curiosity like a child has. Look at things with no attachment and ask yourself: *What is this?* as though you are seeing it for the first time.

Onion Analysis

Let us come back to this analogy of an onion. This is to help you understand the differences between the different types of beliefs and also to ensure that you have the right expectations when doing belief change work. On the surface are our perceptions. Underneath that we have behaviors and behavior-based beliefs. Then, going deeper, we have our values, and finally, our core identity and associated beliefs. Just to clarify, perception is the way in which you notice or understand something, whereas a belief carries a strong conviction about something. You do not have as much attachment to your perceptions as you have to your beliefs. You are much more invested in your beliefs. Changing a perception can be as easy as coming across a new piece of information that renders that perception null and void or shifts it in some way. You can, for instance, have a perception of gooseberries not being nice to eat. Then you taste a gooseberry that is really yummy and just like that you become a connoisseur of gooseberries.

So then we have behaviors and behavior-based beliefs as the next layer. Behaviors can also be reasonably easy to change, provided that they are not a result of eroded identity. If somebody has a phobia of pineapples because they once choked on a pineapple, and their brain generalized that pineapples are a threat, that can be permanently healed in less than 20 minutes using Havening®. In this case, it is a behavioral issue; in other words, they are "doing" this phobia and the belief that goes with it is: *pineapples are dangerous.* However, if a behavior is linked to identity, it needs deeper work and takes longer to resolve. Take, addiction, for example (self-destruction as a result of intense self-loathing). In fact, any form of self-sabotaging behavior, as well as perfectionistic and OCD-type behaviors, are identity-based.

The next layer of the onion is values, which we just discussed.

Finally, we have our core identity, which is all we identify with and believe we are. Whenever you say: *I am*, you are connecting to your identity. This is why it is so unfortunate when people have beliefs such as as: *I am unworthy, I am unlovable, I am not good enough, I am sick, I am a loser, I am a perfectionist, I am not wanted, I am powerless, I am not capable, I am a failure, I am stupid*, and so on. Identity-based beliefs are mostly linked to attachment trauma. But you can also have identity-based beliefs that are based on conditioning. For example, a person who has been told repeatedly that once you turn 30, you put on weight easily may believe: *I am fat because I'm over 30.*

Those *I am* type beliefs are much more challenging to change. This is because when you say, *I am worthless*, for example, your subconscious reads it as this is part of you. If you remove that, there will be this sense of loss because you have removed part of who you are. This is a massive secondary gain for many in terms of chronic health issues. When you identify with your health problem, you will have a really hard time getting rid of it, for example, *I am depressed, I am celiac, I am bipolar, I am autistic, I am a Hashi.* So we must be super aware of what we tell ourselves we are. Saying *I am worthless* or *I am a loser* is the worst thing you can do to yourself, other than actually physically kill yourself. It is extremely damaging, and I describe it as an assassination of the soul.

Identifying Your Limiting Beliefs

1. First, I will ask you to identify as many things you are currently believing as you can. We are going to break this down into a number of areas:
   - Health
   - Family/friends
   - Love/intimacy
   - Career/work
   - Money/wealth
   - Spirituality/inner peace.

2. Here is what I would like you to do next. Take a few deep breaths to be more present in the body. Again, I do not want you to overthink this; let your subconscious mind come to the forefront since it already has all the answers. Start with the category of *Health*. Write *Health* at the top of the page. I will now give you some words to start some sentences, and you will write down intuitively two to four endings to each sentence. Focusing on the area of Health only, write down what comes to mind without overanalyzing.
   - *I am...*
   - *I am not...*
   - *I'm too...*
   - *I do...*
   - *I don't...*
   - *I always get...*
   - *I always feel...*

- *I always do...*
- *I will never...*
- *I have...*
- *I don't have...*
- *I can ...*
- *I can't...*
- *It's hard to...*
- *I'm the sort of person who...*

3. Next, I want you to do this with each of those areas. Same beginning to those sentences, but each time focus on a different area of your life.

Now that you have done this exercise, you have many beliefs written down. Next, we will use a process of belief change that will help you redesign your belief system so that it serves you better.

Belief Change Work Strategies

Next, we are going to look at belief change work. I will give you a process inspired by my colleague, Tony Burgess. He describes his exact approach, which I have adapted slightly, in his book *Beliefs and How to Change Them for Good.* Here, I am giving you the key steps of this technique, which is certainly enough for you to work with and change your limiting beliefs successfully. Remember that quite simply your beliefs are really only your truths until they stop being your truths. Also, remember that if you do not put in your mind what you want to be there, others will do it for you. Imagine that you go to a restaurant, and you are allowing a waiter to tell you what to order. This is the equivalent of what happens to people who are not interested to do this work.

So here are the steps:

1. In the last section, you identified different things you currently believe that relate to those different areas of your life. So the first thing I would like you to do is to write those headings on a piece of paper, ranking them from most to least important.

2. Next, look at the area of your life you have identified as the most important and refer back to all those statements you completed in the previous section in this particular category. These statements, which are essentially your beliefs, need to be sorted into those that serve you and those that do not serve you. You can underline those that do not serve you, for example, or mark them in some other way. Those are going to be the ones you'll want to change, as they get in the way of your life and achieving your goals.

   By the way, if you think you can still add to your list, you can do that at any time and then clear all those limiting beliefs using one of the techniques I am sharing with you. In case you are not sure whether a given belief is helpful or unhelpful, I have some questions for you that you can ask yourself to help you decide. Naturally, you will be able to see that some of your statements have negative focus right away, or you'll feel they have a negative impact on you in some way. But some others you may not be so sure about. So ask yourself these questions:

   a. Is the belief supporting your progress or getting in the way of your progress?

b. Is this belief supporting or hindering your resourcefulness?

c. Is it helping you thrive, or is it keeping you stuck or even moving you further away from your desired outcomes?

3. Now that you have identified which of those beliefs in your most important focus area are limiting you and you want to change, I want you to categorize them into identity-based beliefs and beliefs linked more to perceptions or behaviors. You recognize identity-based beliefs easily because they contain *I am* in them. So, this includes all the statements that start with: *I am..., I am not..., I am too...., I am the sort of person who...*, etc. Most of the other beliefs will be behavior, perception, or experience-based, but this does depend on how you completed the sentences, so just categorize them to the best of your ability.

Now reframe all your limiting, identity-based beliefs and change them into behavior, perception, or experience-based beliefs. This is the first step to create some detachment and make those beliefs less permanent, as is the case when something is connected to your identity. The more transient you can make them sound, the easier it will be to shift them. For example: *I am depressed* is an identity-based belief because it contains *I am* within in it. From the subconscious perspective, *depressed* has become part of who this person is (their identity). This has permanence. If this has been repeated over and over (consolidated), it is going to be more challenging to convince the subconscious to let go of it. This is because it will feel to this person that if they were to let go of it, they would lose part of themselves. They will subconsciously resist letting go of part of who they are, which can make them hold on to this depression (secondary gain).

315

So an example of a reframe to make this less permanent and more transient would be to say: *I am doing this depression right now, but I am taking steps to heal it.* Even though there is still *I am* in this statement, the emphasis is now on *I am doing* versus *I am being* and on moving through this state of depression that the person is experiencing. Another reframe could be: *I am experiencing some depressing times right now, but this too shall pass.*

4. Once you have completed your reframes, pick the first one of your limiting beliefs in this most important category that you are currently working on and write five *what if* type questions that will counter your limiting belief you have just picked. For example, in the case of *I don't have enough drive to make it happen*, you could write:
    - *What if I have more drive than I actually think?*
    - *What if it doesn't take as much drive as I think to make it happen?*
    - *What if it's just a matter of being organized and methodical?*
    - *What if my motivation increases as a result of reading this book?*
    - *What if I could prove to myself that I can do it?*

    Once you have written your questions down, read them out loud a few times and circle the one that resonates with you the most, the one that makes you think: *I actually do believe that is possible.* If you do not have one that resonates, then come up with some more *what if?* questions until you have one you can really connect with.

5. The next step is about accumulating evidence to support the new belief contained in your most helpful *what if?* question. This will satisfy your conscious mind as you turn this

possibility into your new personal truth (a belief). So now write your most powerful positive *what if?* question at the top of a piece of paper. Next, cross out the words *what if* at the beginning of the question, remove the question mark, add the word *because* at the end, and complete the statement. For example, *What if it's just a matter of being organized and methodical?* would become: *It's just a matter of being organized and methodical because whenever I am organized and methodical, I can achieve things quickly and easily.*

Now complete your statement with as much supporting evidence as you can. Generate as many endings as you can think of. It is important to insert some positive emotions into this, such as excitement, for example. Then go through the arguments out loud a number of times, applying Havening Touch°. Repetition and Havening° will help you consolidate your new belief.

6. Now that you have built a strong case to support your new belief, imagine yourself acting out this new belief. Create a mental movie of yourself with this newly formed belief and spend a few minutes playing that in your mind, applying Havening Touch° for maximum result. Be in your body and make the movie vivid and colorful. Feel what you feel, hear what you hear, see what you see, know what you know, and listen to what you are saying to yourself. Again, emotional input and repetition are very important. To change your beliefs and reprogram your subconscious, you need to put yourself in a suggestible state. Lowering your brain wave activity with visualizations and applying Havening° increases your suggestibility and makes this process faster and more successful.

I recommend you go through this belief change process with all the beliefs you want to change. Depending on your list, this could take you a few weeks to complete. That is why I said to start with the area of your life that is the most important to you. After you have completed the process with a few beliefs, do five minutes of Affirmational Havening® (affirmations being the new beliefs) every day to allow them to be consolidated. Be aware that the beliefs of those around you will help you or hinder you. Unconsciously, they can pull you back down.

Your environment has to change accordingly, or it will end up triggering the old patters and reinforcing them. Your environment was what may have conditioned the belief in the first place, so if that new neural pathway you are working on is not yet very strong and the old one is not yet fully dismantled, you can reactivate it by placing yourself in the same environment. If you never change your environment, it will be more challenging to change your beliefs in the first place due to competing neurochemistry. This is just something to be aware of so you can influence your environment accordingly, to go with your new beliefs. You often hear that you cannot get better in the environment that made you sick. That is not only true from the point of view of toxic mold, EMFs, etc.; it also applies to psycho-energetics.

Releasing Limiting Beliefs through Physical Symbolism
I want to share with you another way in which you can transform some of your beliefs.

1. Take a piece of paper, write your limiting beliefs on it, and tear it into pieces.

2. Throw the pieces away, or for a more powerful effect, burn the torn pieces of paper while consciously focusing on releasing the limiting beliefs as you are watching the smoke. Use Havening® and affirm the process of releasing for more impact. In other words, as you are watching your old beliefs burn, you are applying Havening® and repeating: *I release those old limitations now, I am letting go of my old patterns,* etc.

Releasing Limiting Beliefs through Mental Symbolism

1. Sit down, relax, close your eyes, and take a few deeper breaths. Apply Havening® throughout this exercise.

2. Imagine taking a piece of paper and writing your limiting beliefs on it. Now imagine taking each of the limiting beliefs on your list (and associated negative emotions and memories) and placing them one by one into a big box or a casket.

3. Once they are all in there, slam the lid shut and close the latches.

4. Finally, imagine the casket being carried onto a boat, which is then carried out to sea. Imagine it disappearing over the horizon and out of your sight.

Belief Maintenance

Once you have completed the initial few weeks of changing and consolidating your beliefs and you are starting to experience your life change for the better, is that it? Do you consider it done? Can you assume this new belief will forever remain strong and continue to serve you? Unfortunately, no. After you have done the initial work on your beliefs, you need to then maintain them. Why? A couple of reasons. First of all, humans work on the negative bias principle (survival). This means that the human brain connects and acts on negative messages more quickly and easily than the positive ones. Secondly, we are surrounded by negativity. If we do not take major action to counter this, we get bombarded with negative messages constantly.

So if you do not maintain your new shiny positive beliefs by re-enforcing them and do not cut off as much of the negativity that can mess with your new beliefs as you can, your new beliefs will be compromised. This is usually extremely subtle, and you may find yourself in this state I have termed *enlightened unawareness*. You think you are so enlightened now because you have done all this self-development work, so you switch off and become less aware. Meanwhile, all the negative influences around you are eroding your beliefs. You underestimate the power of those negative influences because you feel your new beliefs are so powerful that it does not matter what you expose yourself to. This is a mistake. You need to remain aware, and you need to maintain what you have achieved with regards to belief change.

So How Do You Maintain the Work You Have Done?

1. Continue to do Affirmational Havening® with your key beliefs. Once you have done this most days for the first 6 – 8 weeks, you can go to the maintenance phase, when you do it once or twice per week, depending on how you feel and what is going on in your life.

2. Restrict the influence of mainstream and social media, as discussed previously.

3. Always evaluate all new relationships from the point of view of toxicity, including work ones. If somebody wants to share negative stuff with you, set boundaries. Be firm. You have to say: *Sorry, but I am not interested in talking about that.* If you have issues setting those boundaries, you have to ask yourself what you are scared of. Why are their needs more important than yours? What patterns are you replicating by not setting those boundaries, and why?

To summarize, most of your core beliefs about yourself and the world around you, by which you live your life as an adult, you created or acquired by the age of 6. Think about your possible "truths" at the age of 0 – 6, or even 0 – 12. Would you say that most of it could have been possibly skewed in some way? You can answer this question by observing children at this age and see how much of their truths are aligned with your truths as an adult. But once again, the beliefs sit in your subconscious, so it does not matter that as an adult you consciously think something is silly or unhelpful (e.g., a phobia). If your younger self was convinced of their "truth" at the time of developing or acquiring the belief, that is what got imprinted into your subconscious mind.

Finally, I want to once again emphasize how powerful beliefs are. We know from research that our body behaves differently towards food we believe is good for us, or we like, and food we do not believe is good for us, or we do not like. This is the case even if nutritionally they offer the exact same amount of carbohydrates, protein, fats, fiber, minerals, vitamins, etc. Case studies of people with split personality disorders show that the same person can be severely allergic to something, and the next moment they could be stuffing their face with the same food and be fine. The only difference is, they shifted into a different personality and this personality believes they can eat this particular food without any issues. The other personality believes they are allergic to this food, so they create the physiology of an allergic response (swelling of the throat, difficulty breathing, etc.) that corresponds to that belief. This is yet another example of how your beliefs dictate your biology. So, in the end, the biology you create is mostly up to you, which is why it is so critically important not to be too quick to accept other people's beliefs or generic "truths" as your own. Instead, be discerning and always tune in to what FEELS true for you.

Action points:

1. Go through the value elicitation and hierarchy exercise to ensure you are clear on your values and value conflicts you may have.

2. Identify and categorize your limiting beliefs.

3. Start transforming your limiting beliefs using the strategies offered.

Setting Healthy Boundaries & Building Great Relationships

How to Identify Toxic People & Relationships

Julia grew up in a dysfunctional family. Her father came from an alcoholic family and was abusive towards both her mother and her. Her mother also had unresolved trauma and was not able to take care of herself, or protect her child. Desperate to remove herself from her family home, Julia left at 16 when she met a man who unfortunately turned out to be even worse than her father. He hit Julia regularly. In the end, she was extracted from that relationship by a couple of friends who gave her shelter and threatened her boyfriend with prosecution if he refused to let her go.

Even though all Julia wanted was to be in a loving relationship, inadvertently she kept attracting abusers and reproducing the pattern. Subconsciously, she believed that was all she deserved and she also associated relationships with abuse. As children we do not know any better, so what our parents model to us becomes coded as "normal." This is why it is so easy to repeat the same patterns that we are exposed to as children, no matter how dysfunctional they are. Unfortunately, at this stage of her life, Julia was still unaware that unless she became more conscious and rewired her subconscious programs, she would continue to attract toxic people into her life.

Then she met a man through work with whom she felt she had an instant connection. She decided that this time things were going to be different. The first few months were indeed very promising, and Julia started to secretly hope he really was the one. She was delighted when he started hinting at marriage. They married within a year, but unfortunately, it did not take long for things to take the wrong turn. They went to a party. Julia's now husband would not normally drink hard liquor, but he got strong-armed by his friends to drink a few shots. That made him aggressive, and after they had returned home, he started a trivial argument and he ended up hitting Julia.

She was devastated. What she dreaded the most was happening again. She really thought she had put all the abuse behind her. She cried all night, and the following day, she felt very unwell. She stayed in bed for a few days but was not getting better. Her whole body ached, and she was feeling extremely fatigued. She could barely get through the day. This went on for months, and eventually, one doctor she went to suggested that she may have fibromyalgia, which was then confirmed.

In the meantime, her relationship was going from bad to worse, as her husband was expecting her to satisfy him in the bedroom, which she was now not able to do. Julia's husband was not hiding his disappointment. He said to her that if she was not going to act like a wife, he would get his needs satisfied elsewhere. This was when Julia reached her breaking point.

She approached me to seek support for her condition. She said she needed to get better so that she was able to proceed with the divorce process. We spent a few months addressing her traumas, limiting beliefs, and poor self-worth. Julia was very committed to the work once she understood that her condition was connected to her history of abuse. She may have pushed some of it to the back of her mind, but her body remembered. Within just a few weeks of therapy, Julia was looking back at her life, struggling to understand how she could ever let anybody treat her this way. Each week, she was feeling better and more resilient.

When she announced she wanted a divorce, her husband laughed. He told her not to be stupid and that she would not have it in her to go through with it. But she did have in her. Julia stayed committed to her self-development work and recovered her health. Plus, now that she knew her own worth, she was not going to let just anybody into her life. Julia ended up marring a very loving and caring man and having a healthy baby girl. She finally got exactly what she always wanted.

Good Relationships Originate within

First of all, there is a reason why this chapter on relationships appears later in the book. Simply, there is no point dissecting your relationships and trying to fix them before you have understood and dealt with your own baggage first. This is because of projection, which I briefly mentioned before. If you have not addressed your traumas, limiting beliefs, and poor self-worth, you will always interpret what other people are doing, saying, and how they are acting through the prism of your unresolved issues. You will project your own resulting emotional toxicity onto other people.

There is this saying: *I am not what you think I am. You are what you think I am.* If you feel unworthy, unlovable, undeserving, etc., you will look for the validation of that in other people's behavior. In other words, they will mirror to you how you feel about yourself and they will treat you exactly how you treat yourself. Think about it. If you have no self-respect, why would you expect anybody else to respect you? If you do not accept yourself, why would you expect anybody else to accept you? If you do not love yourself, why would you expect anybody else to love you? You need to be a shining example for people of how to treat you.

On the other hand, when you shine out onto the world self-love, self-acceptance, and self-respect, that is what will come back to you from others. So good relationships originate within. To put this another way, when you respect, accept, and love yourself, you will quite simply not put up with anybody out there disrespecting you and treating you badly. You will not stand for it. It is as simple as that. When you have self-respect, and somebody is refusing to respect you, you have no issues letting them go. I am not suggesting you go around cutting everybody off. We will be splitting all the relationships you have into groups, and you will deal with them slightly differently. But what I am saying is that if after everything we have covered in this book you still continue let somebody treat you poorly, you are the one making that choice. You are not anybody's victim. When you deal with toxic people, you are the one choosing to let them treat you like crap. Or you can choose not to let them do it. It is up to you. It always has been and always will be.

Unfortunately, many people in abusive relationships do not have enough self-awareness. Often, they have been programmed and controlled so they put up with it. It can also be very painful for them to recognize the depth of abuse and hurt that has been inflicted on them by another person. It is almost easier for them to continue being mistreated and live in denial than to actually face reality. In addition, often people stuck in abusive relationships are scared to reach out for help, or they may not believe they can be helped. One of my hypnotherapy teachers used to get people out of cults. It is not easy to break through that programing when somebody this person cares about is constantly lying to them and manipulating them. But since you are here doing this work, you are clearly not in this category.

I also want to acknowledge that relationships are definitely not black and white. We need to respect other people's choices. Just because we look at a relationship as an observer and we think a person needs saving doesn't mean it is appropriate or what they want. In addition, if you believe in reincarnation, you accept that we all know what we are choosing before coming here. We are choosing those experiences. To a soul, an experience is an experience is an experience. That is all. So from this perspective, if a soul coming down here chooses to be in an abusive relationship, who are we to tell that soul they should not have this experience? This is just another consideration for those who are "rescuers." It is a very different thing, of course, if we are actually asked for help or assistance.

Back to our 3D way of looking at relationships. It is true that most people who are toxic to others behave the way they behave due to their unresolved trauma. We want to have some understanding and compassion towards them, but we should not excuse their behavior. This is, again, about separating a person from their behavior. They may not be rotten people; they are just badly damaged, and that makes their behavior rotten and inexcusable. Some people, because of their unresolved traumas, are addicted to punishing others for their misery. That comes from self-loathing. Then, as a result of treating others badly, they develop even more self-loathing because, unless they are psychopaths, they will experience deep shame when they hurt people. They have this internal turmoil, but in those moments when they do something to make another person feel bad, they momentarily feel like they have won. This does not last though, and they feel even more self-loathing afterwards. But again, if we let people like that abuse us, then not only are we destroying ourselves, but we are not helping them either. Sometimes when somebody decides enough is enough, that could be a wake-up call that both sides need.

Ideally, people should feel safe with each other. When that is the case, our social engagement system is activated. If you remember, that is the ventral branch of the vagus nerve, our rest-digest-detoxify-heal response. When you feel safe in the presence of another human being and your ventral vagus nerve is activated, it often feels like there is resonance and synchronicity. There are cues of safety going back and forth between you and the other person, and, of course, the vibrational frequency you emit is pretty high. When there is no resonance or synchronicity, when we do not feel completely safe with somebody, our nervous system immediately flips to fight-or-flight or even the freeze response. Again, there is no such a thing as a little bit safe or a little bit uncomfortable from the point of view of the nervous system. We are either interpreting the cues as safe, in which case we are in the relaxation response, or we do not feel safe, which activates fight, flight, or freeze.

Toxic Relationship Assessment

We are now going to look at the key characteristics of toxic people and toxic relationships. As you are reading through these, think about which relationships in your life these may apply to.

1. All take, no give, a one-sided relationship, the person lacks genuine concern or interest in you and your life.

2. Leaving you feeling drained (mentally, emotionally, physically, energetically); makes you unhappy or uncomfortable in any way.

3. Lack of trust (a relationship without trust is like a car without gas: you can stay in it all you want, but you will not go anywhere).

4. Hostile atmosphere, constant anger, abuse, volatility, aggression, overreaction, unpredictability, yelling or name calling (or anything that makes you feel unsafe).

5. Constant judgment; when criticism is not intended to be helpful but rather to belittle your values, beliefs, and choices and invalidate your feelings.

6. Persistent unreliability.

7. Narcissism (other party's interest in the relationship is driven by how you can serve them) or nonstop demands.

8. Loaded with negative energy.

9. Communication issues; they talk but do not listen.

10. Continuous disrespect; always undermining or diminishing your self-worth, not respecting boundaries.

11. Mutual avoidance.

12. Insufficient support; the other person is not available when you need help, only when they need something from you.

13. The other person tries to control you, manipulate you openly or in a passive-aggressive manner, or gaslight (a powerful form of manipulation that makes you doubt your perception of what is going on).

14. Never-ending drama (but no desire to change), constant challenges, feels like you walk on eggshells, the person ruins holidays and special occasions.

15. Persistent self-betrayal; if you find yourself changing your opinions to please someone else, you are in a damaging relationship.

16. Feelings of unworthiness; like you do not deserve any better.

17. Feelings of entrapment; you stay because you do not see a way out.

18. The person is envious, gossips, or speaks badly about you behind your back.

19. Shortage of autonomy; you do have the right to say NO but do not feel like you can.

20. The other person feels victimized or obsessive, always blaming others, not willing to take responsibility, or has temper tantrums when they do not get what they want.

21. Laced with dishonesty and lies.

22. The person refuses to compromise.

23. Influences you to lower your standards; you slowly begin accepting what was once not acceptable.

24. Things are stagnant; nothing ever gets resolved.

25. The other person brings out the worst in you; you are unable to be your best self around them.

26. You cannot do anything right; they are always right, and you are always wrong.

27. The other person finds the worst in everything and everyone.

28. Questions and statements become traps and are designed to "catch you out."

29. The person feels and acts entitled without consideration for other people's needs; rules do not apply to them.

30. The person rarely apologizes, and if they do, it is shallow, coerced, or fake.

31. The person undermines your other relationships.

32. The person creates so much stress, anxiety, and pain that your health, ability to work, or general wellbeing are negatively impacted.

Generally, the more of those feel true, the more toxic the relationship. The person in question may be a narcissistic sociopath or they may be simply damaged by life with their behavior being shaped by their unresolved traumas. It is up to you to decide how much toxicity you want to put up with in your relationship. Like I said, if your self-worth is strong, you will not put up with any. People will have to shape up or you part ways with them. However, there are unique situations, and depending on the circumstances, sometimes you may want to make allowances. As long as you are aware and it is your choice, that is fine. Just be careful not to have the relationship erode your self-worth over time. Inviting just a bit of toxicity into your relationship, or shall I say, putting up with it, will work much like allowing a bit of toxic media into your life. We have talked about it. Bit by bit, it will have that destructive effect, but because it is a drip effect, you will probably not notice until your identity has been eroded and you feel more fearful, guilty, ashamed, less confident, etc.

The Art of Boundary Setting

When deciding how to deal with toxic relationships in your life, it helps to categorize your relationships into groups:

- people you have no emotional attachment to (e.g., co-workers, social media "friends")

- people you have some attachment to (e.g., more distant friends or family)

- people you feel emotionally attached to right now, such as close friends and family.

You may have already started setting better boundaries as a result of the work you have done so far. The moment your self-acceptance, self-respect, self-trust, and self-love increase, you will almost automatically start pulling away from some toxic people and say *no* to behaviors that are no longer acceptable to you. When you increase your self-worth, you increase your dominant vibrational frequency. Plus, you now operate from a different subconscious program, which means that your expression and behavior changes. When your vibration increases, you stop resonating with certain people and behaviors that you previously accepted without questioning. So the other person is now facing a choice. They can either try to stay the same as before. I say *try* because soon enough, they realize that their old way of operating is not producing the same results as before. Or they can adapt their behavior to this new situation.

This will happen predominantly at the subconscious level. This can mean that they may be trying to push your buttons harder, being more aggressive, etc. If you stay true to yourself, this will not work, and they will probably end up in turmoil. Or they can shape up and adjust their behavior to match the level you are now at. If they do not, the relationship is over. I hope you can see how this works. This will happen over a longer period of time because people rarely change in an instant. They usually play this ping-pong game. Again, a lot of it will be subconscious. Either way, eventually, if the other person does not adjust to the changes the first person is going through, the relationship will not survive. So basically, if you want to change other people, you can do it by changing yourself, your own vibration, programs, behavior, and responses. Simply, if you change, they cannot stay the same. It will not work.

Strategies for Setting Healthy Boundaries

Let me now share with you some tips and strategies for dealing with your relationships that fall into those three groups. When you deal with the first group, people you have not got much of an emotional connection with, the first thing to do is to decide which of these relationships you want to work on and which you can just let go of right away. If you have difficulties letting some of these relationships go, you need to ask yourself why. If you have toxic relationships with people you are not even that connected to and yet you are scared to just bin them, then you have much more self-worth work to do. On the other hand, when you can say: *I used to put up with your nonsense but I am not going to do that anymore!*, then you know you are really getting somewhere.

Regardless of which group a relationship falls into, one of the things you need to do is to set better boundaries. Boundaries are a way to take care of ourselves. When we set boundaries, we are less angry and resentful because we ensure that our needs are getting met. Boundaries are about making our expectations clear so other people know what to expect from us and how we want to be treated. People are more likely to respect our boundaries when we communicate them clearly. As I've said, some people will do everything they can to resist our efforts to set boundaries. They will argue, scream and shout, blame, ignore, manipulate, threaten, or want to physically hurt us. And while we cannot really prevent people from acting like this, we can learn to set clear boundaries and take care of ourselves. The stronger your self-worth, the easier this will be.

There are three parts to setting boundaries.

1. Identify your boundaries. Be clear about what you are trying to achieve before trying to communicate or enforce the boundary.

2. Communicate your boundaries or expectations clearly, calmly, and consistently. It is really important to stick to the facts without overexplaining, blaming, or becoming defensive. Stay true to yourself and stay calm and matter-of-fact

when communicating your boundaries. If that is challenging, use the tools I have already shared with you to deal with being triggered so you can be successful. If you are making a request, be specific so that both sides know exactly what they are agreeing to.

When I set boundaries with somebody, I state it in a way that there is no discussion or debate. I simply inform them what is going to happen while remaining calm. Tonality is very important here. You can use whatever words you want, but if your tonality says you are not convinced yourself about what you are doing, you will not have a result. This is why you need to believe that you deserve to be treated with respect. What you believe and feel inside matters. You must be congruent, or else the other side will pick up on the conflicting signals. You can use gentle words, but they must be communicated in a way that leaves no doubt you are not going to shift your position.

3. If your boundaries are not respected, evaluate your options and take appropriate action. If you explained your position and you are still getting nowhere, you need to dissect it and figure out why. You may have to let the relationship go. Sometimes that is the only thing you can do.

Dealing with Chronic Boundary Violators

I am now going to share with you some ideas that can help you choose the best approach for dealing with chronic boundary violators.

1. Decide whether the boundary you are trying to enforce is negotiable.

Some boundaries are more important than others. Identifying what you are willing to put up with and what you consider unacceptable or non-negotiable will help you decide if you may be willing to compromise. Compromise can be a positive choice IF both people are adjusting. I advise that you do not just compromise yourself and what you believe in if the other person is doing nothing to help the relationship. You will only end up building resentment if you do that. True compromise is not about abandoning your needs to please someone else. If someone repeatedly violates boundaries that are important to you, ask yourself how long you are willing to put up with such behavior.

2. Be consistent.

It is challenging to repeatedly set the same boundary with someone who is not receptive. What can happen is that in this situation you start to give in and become inconsistent with your boundaries. It helps to write down what is happening. Record the boundary violations and your responses so you can analyze them and check for weaknesses. If you notice that you are not consistent, make adjustments. If you are being consistent, writing things down can help you get clarity about what you are willing to accept and where it may help you to tweak what you are doing. That said, once you have figured out your limits, you HAVE to be consistent. Only make threats you can 100 percent follow through with. For example: *If you don't respect this boundary I have set, I will leave.* If you just say it and do not do it, you will have zero credibility. Boundaries should not be a way to punish or control someone else. As we said, boundaries are a way to take care of yourself. However, there are consequences to violating someone's boundaries and, at times, issuing a warning or threat is absolutely called for. Just make sure you can execute it.

3. Practice detachment.

When you are in a state of fear, it is understandable that you want to control things to protect yourself. When you are in a situation where your boundaries are being chronically violated and for whatever reason you are not in a position to cut off the relationship, detachment can help you preserve your sanity. Detaching does not mean you do not care about this person; it just means you are taking care of your own mental and physical health. The best way to detach is to deal with your own emotional responses so that the other person's behavior does not trigger you anymore, but you can also detach by:

- physically leaving a dangerous or uncomfortable situation and simply refusing to spend time with this person
- altering your response, e.g., instead of taking something personally or yelling, you can shrug off a rude comment or make a joke of it (this is an example of how you make people adjust their behavior by adjusting yours)
- letting the person deal with the consequences of the choices and decision they make
- choosing not to give advice or participate in the same old arguments.

4. Accept that some people will not respect your boundaries no matter what you do.

This can be disappointing to realize when you believe that the other person should care enough to respect your boundaries. However, at some point, you may need to decide whether you want to continue the relationship. Essentially, you can choose to accept their behavior or you can choose to disengage. Sometimes the only way to protect yourself is to stop associating with toxic people who do not respect you. Again, this is not about punishing others. Limited or no-contact is a form of self-care. If someone is hurting you physically or emotionally, you owe it to yourself to act on that. You are not obliged to have a relationship with anyone who makes you feel bad about yourself. That includes family members. Family and friends should lift you up and support you, not leave you depressed, anxious, angry, ashamed, or confused.

5. If necessary, get support.

If you are in a toxic relationship that is abusive or dangerous, please reach out for support from friends, family members, your spiritual community, myself, or whoever else you are comfortable approaching.

Overall, the hardest thing to do will be to set boundaries with people who you are close to and have a strong emotional connection with, like your closest family or our partner. It is essential to recognize any toxicity in your relationship with your parents. Parents can absolutely abuse their adult children if emotional baggage has not been addressed. These relationships are more challenging to call out and deal with because of what I already said about the inner conflict many people have. On the one hand, we want our parents' acceptance, but on the other, we may harbor resentment or anger towards them if they have harmed us in any way. Many people do not want to admit to themselves that their relationship with their mother and/or their father is toxic because it may be painful for them to face and address that reality.

Again, if your self-worth work is not done and your inner child still feels wounded, you will struggle to call your relationship with your parents out because your inner child is still crying for Mom's and Dad's approval. In this case, they may be still disrespecting or abusing you in some way, may be taking advantage of your kindness, and you will just go along with it. But inside you will be building up resentment and feeling miserable. On the other hand, people who identify toxicity in their parental relationships and take action to resolve it usually find this extremely liberating. I have had many clients over the years who can attest to that.

The most important thing when it comes to any relationship is that we do honor ourselves and our own needs. This is why we must set healthy boundaries when dealing with our parents. Without proper boundaries, parents may believe and feel that it is OK to impose their beliefs and ways of living onto their adult children. But again, you need to figure out what works for you first and then communicate it clearly. If you are not clear on what you need them to do or not to do, you will not be able to communicate this successfully and it will not work. Be clear, concise, assertive, and repetitive. You may sound like a "broken record" until they accept that they need to change their behavior, but that is OK. You continue to repeat your needs clearly and concisely over and over. This demonstrates that you are sticking to your decisions and are not interested in engaging in an argument or negotiation about your boundaries. Some people may choose to cut the ties with their parents altogether. This is usually if parents were or still are offenders or abusers and the person decides they do not want anything to do with them. They may have tried different ways to try to set boundaries and the parent(s) continued to violate them so they end up "divorcing" their parents. They need to do a lot of inner child and acceptance work but there is no reason why this should not work for people if they feel this is the only way.

Setting boundaries in our intimate relationships is also very important. As we know, many people do not attach securely in childhood, and if they start having relationships before they heal their insecure attachment, which obviously happens all the time because nobody teaches this at school, then they will end up in relationships they are not happy in. We see many relationships between ambivalents and avoidants, which tend not to work out very well because, at the core, these two attachment styles have opposing approaches to intimacy. People with the ambivalent attachment style move towards intimacy as that is their dominant need, whereas avoidants move away from intimacy to reclaim their space and maintain their independence. There is this constant cycle of: ambivalent wants to be close, avoidant runs away, ambivalent starts a fight, avoidant avoids a solution. This is followed by a short-lived reconciliation, and then they go off again.

When you have two ambivalents getting together, this match usually ends badly and quickly, as neither partner is good at anticipating the needs of the other. It is not impossible for two ambivalents to bond and learn to satisfy each other's security needs, but it is rare. Similarly, two avoidants in a relationship is a pretty disastrous combination and is actually quite rare. Without a partner willing to do some of the communication work, this couple type rarely even gets going. The *why bother?* attitude from both of them tends to end the relationship quickly under even a minor stress. So, most commonly, we see an ambivalent-avoidant, and then secure-avoidant, secure-ambivalent, and secure-secure combination. Obviously, if we have two secure people in a relationship, it is going to be a happy and healthy relationship with great communication, so no problems here. In those other situations, if one partner is more secure, they can actually help the other person shift to a more secure attachment, but if the person does no self-development work, they will forever have to be reassured. A secure partner can help but they cannot do all the work for the other person.

Other Considerations for Building Great Relationships

Working on your self-worth and setting healthy boundaries is not just important when dealing with toxic people. It is also important when we want to build great relationships. Having strong self-worth will ensure that you attract the right people into your life in the first place, and communicating your boundaries clearly from the start can prevent many unnecessary conflicts. But there are also other things I encourage you to consider if you want your relationships to be great. One of them is effective communication.

How to Communicate More Effectively

1. I encourage you to always own what you say, do, think and feel. Not stating things as facts or pointing the finger and blaming goes a long way towards improving how we communicate with others. You can eliminate much of that by making sure you avoid sweeping generalizations and do not overuse the verb *to be* in all its forms. I am not talking about people who start every sentence with *I am*. I am talking about making statements about things as though they are set in stone and are ultimate truths. For example, when you

341

state: *Red is the best color*, you are likely to get an immediate pushback from whoever you are talking to, and they might say: *No, it isn't. Blue is the best color.* Or, if you say something like: *They are bad people*, you might get a push back and have somebody objecting: *No they are not!* It does not matter what the subject of the conversation is. When you say: *it is, they are, she is, he is, you are*, etc., it sounds like you are stating a fact. This is essentially a shortcut to alienating people and a recipe for how to lose rapport with somebody right away. You cannot successfully navigate relationships without being able to stay in rapport. The more sensitive the subject, the worse the consequences will be, including heated arguments.

The solution to this is very simple. It requires you to be more aware and own whatever you say, do, think, or feel. Use phrases such as: *In my personal opinion..., I personally feel/think..., My sense is...*, etc. If you say: *In my opinion, red is the best color*, all the other person can really say is: *I disagree. For me it is blue.* That is fine. Now you both know where you stand, and you can respect each other's opinions. The other person will not feel like you are telling them how they should perceive the world, so their reaction will be completely different. This is a very powerful way of communicating and can diffuse a lot of conflict.

2. There is another language trick to be aware of. This is the use of *but* versus *and*. Whenever you use these joining words, you have two parts to the sentence. Just remember that when you use *but* to join two parts of a sentence, you essentially delete the first part. This is what your subconscious mind will hear. So use these words in a mindful way. When you say to somebody, for example: *I love you, but it bothers me*

when you tell me what to do, all they are hearing is what comes after the *but*. The fact that you said *I love you* first is not being heard. That gets deleted. All they will hear is the criticism that comes after the *but*. So if you want somebody to pay more attention and be more responsive, you might want to say: *I love you, and I would love it if you allowed me to decide for myself without telling me what to do*. On the other hand, we can use *but* to acknowledge somebody's concern while making it less of a concern, for example, *I know you are uneasy about this, but everything will be OK*. You acknowledge they are uneasy, then you delete it with *but* and you make their subconscious mind focus on *everything will be OK*.

3. Avoid *should-ing* on people unless they specifically ask for it. Most people do not take kindly to being told what to do.

4. Avoid stereotyping and promoting *us versus them* thinking, language, and actions. Also, do not assume that all the people who have a certain view hold the same exact position. If you seek to identify gradation and distinctions in people's beliefs or practices, you have more of a chance to find some common ground. Even if somebody has an opposing position, looking for anything you can actually agree with, rather than focusing on differences, will result in a much more successful communication.

5. It is very healthy to mentally swap roles with people to examine things from the other person's perspective and also to imagine how someone else may be viewing your ideas.

6. It is good to share why you have come to believe what you believe and also encourage others to do the same. Not everybody is mature enough to participate in this exercise, but

343

you can end up having really great, enlightening debates with those who are.

7. Besides what the person is saying, pay attention to how they describe things, their body language, and their tonality. One golden rule of successful communication is to listen twice as much as you talk. Everybody is familiar with this concept, yet look at how many people fail to apply it. It is also very healthy to ask questions to clarify your understanding, but when asking questions, be sure you listen to the answer.

8. Most people have more in common than they think. We have been artificially conditioned to believe we are different. This suits the corrupt elites. The more humanity is divided, the easier we are to control. When people connect at the human level, they usually discover that they are more similar than different. Keep this in mind when dealing with others and try to uncover the hidden connections between you and other people.

Physical, Verbal & Tonal Cues

You may be already aware that verbal cues (words) account for only 7 percent of our communication. Even though the words themselves do matter, our physiology is the biggest contributor to communication (gestures, posture, blinking, breathing, facial expressions) at 55 percent. Think about the difference in people's face when they are angry and tense and when they are happy (smiling, eyes wide and bright). People read your gaze and facial expressions all the time, even if they are not conscious of it. The second biggest chunk in our communication is tonality (pace, pitch, volume, tone, pauses, etc.) at 38 percent of the communication pie chart. So be mindful of your tone of voice.

How we use our voice, especially the prosody, or tone of voice, communicates safety or danger to others. A melodic voice promotes a sense of safety, whereas a monotone or robotic voice is usually perceived as cold, uncaring, and in some cases, threatening. So you may want to pay attention to how you modulate your voice when speaking with others. Shrill, booming, screeching tones will trigger our survival responses. Calming, soothing, well-modulated voices will reduce a sense of threat in people. That will make interactions more successful and productive. Apart from communicating with our physiology, words, and tonality, we obviously also communicate energetically, whereby our resonance is picked up by other people.

Utilizing Transactional Analysis

We have previously talked about TA from the point of view of understanding our own psyche. We were considering how our Child, Parent, and Adult ego states interact together and how that can lead to having internal conflicts and also how we can create more internal calm when we heal our Child and make our Parent more nurturing. I now want to briefly look at how we can use TA to improve our interactions with people. This is predominantly what TA is used for. When two people communicate, each exchange is called a transaction. Many of our problems and stress come from transactions that are unsuccessful. There are different types of transactions: Parallel (Complementary), Crossed, Hidden (Ulterior), which are essentially psychological games.

COMPLEMENTARY TRANSACTIONS

In this case, individuals respond as expected. This happens when you address someone's Child ego state from your Parent ego state, for example. Or it could be the Adult addressing the Adult. Either way, they respond as expected, so the exchange goes back and forth until: a) someone breaks the cycle by coming from a different ego state; b) the person feels they have made their point; c) one or both parties have received what in TA we call the "strokes" (attention) they need.

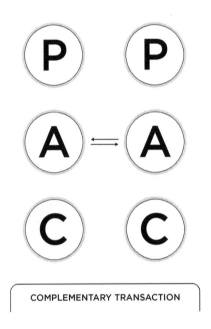

COMPLEMENTARY TRANSACTION

For example:

Person A (Parent ego state): *You still haven't given me the report I asked you for. You're always doing this.*

Person B (Child ego state): *It wasn't my fault!*

Person A (Parent ego state): *It's never your fault. So, who's to blame this time?*

Person B (Child ego state): *I wasn't given the data by accounts.*

Person A (Parent ego state): *You should have asked them for the data.*

Person B (Child ego state): *I did, but they were making excuses why they could not do it right away.*

CROSSED TRANSACTIONS

In this case, a person's particular ego state is addressed, but they come from a different ego state, which is different to the one "expected" by the initiator. Because of this, crossed transactions tend to come to an end sooner than parallel transactions.

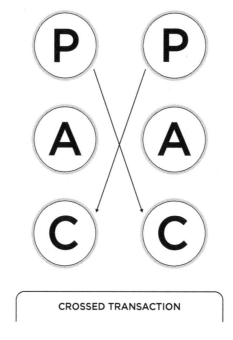

CROSSED TRANSACTION

Example 1:

Person A (Parent ego state addressing the other person's Child ego state): *You still haven't given me the report I asked you for. You're always doing this.*

Person B (responding from Parent rather than Child ego state): *If you were as critical of the accounts department as you are of me, then maybe I would get the information I asked them for.*

Person A has to change tack now because they subconsciously know that if they continue to address this other person's Child ego state, they are going to get push back. Essentially, they are not getting the outcome they wanted. They subconsciously approached the situation as a critical parent scolding a child, but the other person is not having any of it. This is an example how YOU can control other people's behavior. Simply do not let them manipulate you the way they always have done. If you are aware of which ego state they are addressing, respond from a different one (preferably Adult). You will throw them off, and they will HAVE to adjust their communication.

Example 2:
Person A (Parent ego state addressing the other person's Child ego state): *You still haven't given me the report I asked you for. You're always doing this.*

Person B (responding from Adult rather than Child ego state): *Yes. I understand the problem and I would appreciate your help in getting the last information I need from the accounts department.*

Again, if person A keeps addressing this other person like a child when they are responding from their adult, they are going to look like a complete idiot, so they will have to pull back now.

HIDDEN TRANSACTIONS
Hidden (ulterior) transactions are the ones which appear to be straightforward communications but which actually contain

an unspoken message that carries with it a hidden agenda. It is these transactions which mostly lead to games being played (often seen in personal relationships). With ulterior transactions there is a hidden hook which pulls us into a game if we are not aware of what is happening. Below is an example. We will assume that this relationship is already strained.

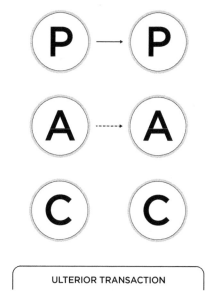

ULTERIOR TRANSACTION

Person A: *Have you seen the car keys?*

This in itself is an innocent question, but let us say that because there is already tension in the relationship, there is an undertone to this message (i.e.: *You had the keys last, and they are not where they should be!*).

So it may appear on the surface like this is a person operating from their Adult addressing the other person's Adult ego state. But in reality, their tonality and body language indicate that they are in their critical Parent addressing this person's Child ego state. If Person B ignores the passive aggressive undertone and responds from their Adult, they may be able to end this exchange without an argument. However, it is likely that the other person will probably find something else to be passive aggressive or even openly aggressive about. If on the other hand, person who is being addressed gets sucked in as they are subconsciously detecting this criticism and they respond from their Child, some sort of an argument or sulking is almost certain. So essentially these ulterior transactions involve two ego states simultaneously.

Another example of this would be an exchange between a sneaky salesman and a buyer:

Salesman: *This car is superior, but it is beyond most people's reach.*

On the surface, they are addressing the buyer's Adult from their Adult, casually stating a fact. However, on a different level their Adult is actually addressing the buyer's Child, saying: *This car is superior, but you can't have it because it is expensive and you can't afford it.* So now the buyer can indeed respond from their Adult, saying: *Yes, you are right, this car is superior, but it is beyond my reach.* Or they can fall for the manipulation, depending on how insecure they are, and respond from their Child: *This is the one I want, and this is the one I will have.* That is, of course, what the salesman is counting on.

So, hopefully, you can see how this works. When you are aware which ego state in you are in at any given time, and you can recognize which ones people are really in, which means interpreting not just the words but also tonality, body language, etc., you can navigate relationships much more successfully.

Social Connection Versus Social Anxiety

To end this chapter, I want to mention social connection. You may have heard about the link between feeling socially isolated and mortality. That connection is stronger than the link between factors such as hypertension, air pollution, physical inactivity, alcohol consumption, smoking, and mortality! There are many studies that have pointed to lack of social connection having a negative impact on health and mortality rates. Much of this evidence has come out from studying the Blue Zones. Researchers looking at those different places around the world, where many people live into their 90s and 100s, have identified a number of factors that contribute to these people's longevity. One of those key factors is social connection. So why is that? For most people, not having social connection is emotionally toxic. That toxicity comes from internal stress linked to lacking a feeling of belonging, lacking engagement with others, or having deficiencies in terms of meaningful relationships. People may socially isolate as a result of physical or mental health issues, economic factors, or withdrawal as a result of experiencing loss.

When you feel good and safe with somebody, you release oxytocin. Oxytocin is known as the "love hormone" because of its important role in the formation and maintenance of mother-child bonding and also sexual attachments. In fact, researchers have discovered that oxytocin released through any type of connection triggers the release of serotonin. In a chain reaction, the serotonin then activated the *reward circuitry* of the nucleus accumbens, resulting in a happy feeling. Remember that Havening® triggers oxytocin. However, what I want you to be careful of is not to fall into this trap of being obsessive about your social connection just because researchers say you must be socially connected to be healthy. We should not generalize this. Why?

It is true that humans are social creatures and we have evolved to be with others, but how do we know if we are scoring health points in terms of this social connection and when we have a deficiency in this area? Again, this all has to do with the nervous system response. When you hear that social connection is good for your vagus nerve, it is a sweeping generalization that shows a lack of understanding of how this works. Social connection is only good for you if your internal response to it is positive and you feel safe, and therefore, your social nervous system (i.e., your ventral vagus nerve) is activated.

If you feel anxious about interacting with people, if the thought of having to interact with somebody causes you anxiety, or the interactions you have with people are not enjoyable, or you feel annoyed, irritable, etc., then you enter one of the survival states, which has the opposite effect on your nervous system. Many people feel they should be more sociable because we are conditioned this way, but it does not really work for them.

It is important to be honest with yourself. If you avoid people because you suffer from social anxiety and you keep saying you are fine on your own but deep inside you wish you had more friends, or you wish you felt more connected to something, you need to act on this. Hopefully, by now you have dealt with some of your traumatic memories and limiting beliefs, and you are starting to feel more and more empowered, worthy, and deserving. However, if your time spent alone is not productive, or is still stressful in any way, then you need to revisit those aspects of psycho-energetic healing so you can address this problem fully.

Equally, you may be one of those people who is happy being on your own. You may have a couple of friends, or a partner, and that is it. Does this mean you are damaging your health? If this is what you enjoy and you are genuinely happy with that, then of course not. That is absolutely fine. Not everybody is going to be super sociable. Many people who are empaths get drained by interacting with people and they are much happier when they are on their own. Monks who have limited social contact do not get sick. Quite the opposite. They are healthy people. Most of their connection is a spiritual connection. As they feel spiritually connected, they also tend to put a lot of emphasis on everything and everyone being one. If you are connected to yourself and to Source, you are connected to everything in the universe. They are peaceful and at ease with that knowing. So no, we do not have to have many people around us to be healthy. Many people choose quality of their connections over quantity, and that is the right way to go about it. It is all about how meaningful the connections that you do have are.

So the best thing to do is to ask yourself: how connected do you feel? Let your heart give you the answer. Maybe you have animals and you feel connected to them. Maybe you are very spiritual and you feel connected to Source. Is that enough? If it makes you feel good and you are happy, it is absolutely enough. Meaningful social connection is definitely NOT about the size of your social network. You can have hundreds of friends and feel lonely. Just consider the fakeness of most so-called connections people have on social media. Most of it is the opposite of connection. It is fake and toxic. Social media and other modern-day factors are reducing face-to-face social connectedness, which actually exacerbates feelings of perceived social isolation.

A national analysis conducted by researchers at the University of Pittsburgh School of Medicine found that young adults in the U.S. who use social media more frequently than their peers report higher levels of perceived social isolation! So this is purely and simply about your internal interpretation of how socially connected you feel. When asking yourself how connected, cared for, and valued you feel, think more broadly. Think about people, animals, nature, universe, your higher self, the Creator. What else needs to fall into place in your life, or what else do you need to do to feel optimally connected?

Action points:

1. Using the Toxic Relationship Assessment, identify people in your life you have toxic relationships with.

2. Categorize your problematic relationships into the three groups discussed and consider what boundaries you need to set in order for those relationships to serve you better and be more conducive to health and healing.

3. Consider your most common relationship problems, misunderstandings, or arguments from the point of view of TA. Analyze which ego states are at play in those situations, what sorts of transactions they are, and how you could improve those common issues by responding from a different ego state.

Addressing Energetic Aspects of Healing & Biofield Optimization

Understanding Our Energetic Anatomy & Setting Energetic Boundaries

Janet got diagnosed with breast cancer shortly after her 52nd birthday. She approached me for support right at the beginning of her healing journey. Janet used to work as a nurse but left the conventional healthcare system in her forties, as she disagreed with much of what she was witnessing on a daily basis. In fact, she admitted she no longer had much faith in conventional medicine or the traditional treatments they offered to cancer patients.

The main reason she approached me in the first place was to help her manage stress. She experienced being shouted down to by everyone around her. Somehow her family, friends, and doctors pretended they knew what was right for her better than she did. Janet wanted to go down the naturopathic route, but nobody was prepared to listen to what she wanted. Janet found it very difficult to assert herself. She had never been able to put her foot down and defend her position, but this was her health and possibly her life at stake, so it was now or never.

Naturally, her inability to assert herself stemmed from childhood trauma. Both of her parents were narcissistic and the adaptation she developed in order to feel safe and be even remotely accepted by her parents was to please. Apart from lacking self-confidence, Janet lacked self-nurturing and self-appreciation. She would continuously take care of others and ignore herself. She never felt loved as a child so, of course, as an adult she felt unlovable. She carried unhealthy guilt and shame. Janet understood that in order to heal, apart from addressing her biochemistry, she needed to do deep emotional and energetic work and she was ready to do that.

She decided to go to a natural health clinic in Germany, specializing in cancer care, and we continued to work remotely. We focused on belief and trauma work, on her attachment trauma, in particular. I got her to do specific heart chakra balancing work and visualize her ideal outcome daily. I also advised that she should work with an energy healer. Janet chose to have her progress assessed with thermography, and after the first four weeks of treatments at the clinic and the psycho-energetic work, the cancer stopped progressing. Janet was very pleased and optimistic, as when she was first diagnosed, she had been told to expect the cancer would continue to progress. The following two months of combining all these natural therapeutic approaches brought further good news, as her thermography results looked even better.

Janet felt good and for the first time in her life felt truly excited about living and the future. She started socializing again, and it was at one of her social outings that she met somebody. He was a very interesting man who recently had a spiritual awakening. It was an instant connection. Because all the self-development work Janet had done by that point, she felt more lovable and was now open to receiving love! As her relationship started to blossom, her cancer continued to disappear. Janet believed that inviting love into her life was what completed her recovery. That and becoming much more spiritual. Within a year, she was free of cancer and planning her wedding. Her thermography results not only showed she was free of cancer but that she was now *low cancer risk*. At the start, all Janet's challenges were characteristic of an imbalanced heart chakra, so it is not surprising that learning to love herself and accepting love as something she was worthy of had such a big impact on her healing.

It Is All about Frequencies

As we said previously, all matter is made up of energy. Everything in the universe moves and vibrates constantly. Nothing rests. Anybody who tries to fight that universal fact will struggle to heal. Anybody who tries to only address their health and healing from the point of view of physicality and biochemistry will not get even remotely close to tapping into their actual healing potential. Most people are kept in the dark about their true potential for healing, as we know, and do not realize what is actually possible. Even if they accept that emotions play a role in healing but neglect the energy field, they will still be limiting what they can achieve.

Obviously, as we already said, thoughts, emotions, and beliefs are actually energy, so by addressing those we are already working energetically. But I am talking about going beyond that and addressing specific energetic imbalances in our biofield. The biofield should be, and I believe in the future will be, recognized as a key aspect of our health and well-being. Chronic disruptions in our energy field lead to disease eventually, as those disruptions affect all the different bodies (mental, emotional, physical). The physical body is the last to break down, not the first like many people have been conditioned to think. Also, as I said before, disruptions in our biofield also create more potential for those dense states of consciousness like fear, anger, sadness, depression, anxiety, and so on.

Just to clarify, there are many energy fields. These include the physically measurable electromagnetic and magnetic fields generated by all living cells, tissues, and organs and the human body as a whole. There are also subtle fields emanating from all pulsing units of life. The reality is that the body is a series of electromagnetic processes, rather than just chemical ones, and the body's bioenergetic fields impact our health. Electromagnetic fields are created when electric currents flow. Just like what happens when you turn on the lights in your house. Our bioenergetic system is made up of magnetic fields throughout the body. Our organs generate electrical currents that flow through tissues and therefore generate magnetic fields both within and around the body.

The brain is constantly sending electrical signals and the heart has the most powerful electromagnetic field in the body. The heart's electrical field is about 60 times greater in amplitude than the electrical activity generated by the brain. And the magnetic field produced by the heart is more than 100 times greater in strength than the field generated by the brain. This magnetic field can be detected up to three feet away from the body. What is also very important is the concept of coherence.

Coherence is when two waves and their frequencies match up to one another. We want our brains and hearts to be in coherence because that promotes healing. When we feel positive emotions, love gratitude, we produce coherent waves. When we feel anger, fear, jealousy, etc., we produce incoherent waves. The more we embody coherent expression, the better our body functions.

The nervous system is an electrical system within the body, a network of over seven trillion nerves. These nerves are continually firing messages back and forth between the body and the brain. We have previously mentioned brain waves, which is basically all about electromagnetic flow. The frequency of a brain wave determines what process it creates in the brain. The bottom line is that we are electric. When somebody's heart stops, they will use electricity to try to bring the heart back online.

This flow of information (energy) can be disrupted by many things, including: negative thoughts, chemical toxins, EMFs, biological agents, etc.

Every living thing has its own frequency that is unique to them, much like a thumbprint. This natural frequency in every living thing is called a resonant frequency. Every tissue and organ has its own frequency, so your heart, your liver, your blood cells, etc. all have different resonant frequencies that are optimal for them. Again, when that optimal resonance is disrupted, this opens us up to disease. When we are talking about healing from the energetic perspective, we are talking about optimizing energy flow but also about attracting healing energy and repulsing damaging energy. This is what the field of bioenergetics is about, and there are endless therapeutic modalities that utilize these principles, such as acupuncture, bioresonance technology, homeopathy, flower remedies, sound healing, Reiki, Jin Shin Juytsu, hypnotherapy, grounding, crystal therapy, and many others that are great for helping us heal chronic conditions.

It is important to emphasize that the body's electromagnetic field extends outside of the physical body. This is a difficult concept for some because this is something that most people cannot see. Some can, of course. Most people can feel when their field is being interfered with, but they do not think about it in this way. When a stranger gets too close to you, you may instinctively pull away and feel like your space has been invaded. That is because they entered your energy field. Even though you may not be able to see it at this time, you can feel it.

I want to talk a bit more about our energetic field anatomy now, based on the work of Barbara Ann Brennan, a very gifted spiritual healer and teacher, and some others.

Our Energetic Anatomy

Scientists have been investigating the existence of the human energy field that surrounds our entire body for over a hundred years, adding to the knowledge our ancestors already possessed. This field consists of multiple bands of energy called auric layers or auric fields. This is our subtle body, which connects us to the outside world. If you could see it (some people can), you would see the biophotons that Fritz-Albert Popp proved existed back in the early 70s. These photons are particles of colored light (quanta) that the human body emits. This is basically what we call the aura. There are seven subtle layers, or bodies, in the auric system. You can think of them as layers of an onion. Auric fields connect to the chakras, unifying what happens inside and outside of a person. The seven subtle bodies hold various forms of information and correspond to the chakra system.

1. Physical field (body) is lowest in frequency and regulates the physical body.

2. Etheric field (body) is the blueprint for the physical body that it surrounds (extends ¼ inch to 2 inches from the physical body).

3. Emotional field (body) regulates our emotional state (extends 1 to 3 inches from the body).

4. Mental field (body) processes ideas, thoughts, and beliefs (extends 3 to 8 inches from the body).

5. Astral field (body) is a connection between the physical and spiritual realms (extends a foot from the physical body).

6. Etheric template body exists only on the spiritual plane, holds our highest ideals for existence, and is only visible to advanced healers and clairvoyants (extends about 1.5 feet from the body).

7. Celestial field (body) accesses universal energies and it is experienced as spiritual love, joy, elation, and bliss (extends about 2.5 feet from the body).

8. Causal field (body) resembles an egg which pulsates and vibrates at high speeds and surrounds and protects everything within it (extends about 4 feet from the body). This field is a reflection of everything your soul has undergone and is your connection to Source and accepting your oneness with the universe.

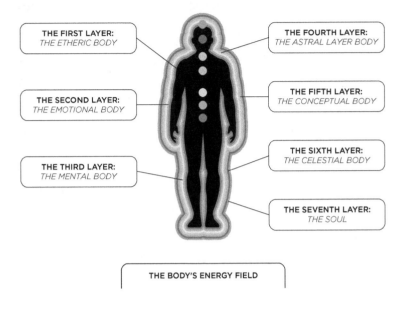

THE FIRST LAYER:
THE ETHERIC BODY

THE SECOND LAYER:
THE EMOTIONAL BODY

THE THIRD LAYER:
THE MENTAL BODY

THE FOURTH LAYER:
THE ASTRAL LAYER BODY

THE FIFTH LAYER:
THE CONCEPTUAL BODY

THE SIXTH LAYER:
THE CELESTIAL BODY

THE SEVENTH LAYER:
THE SOUL

THE BODY'S ENERGY FIELD

The aura has been known by many names in various cultures. Christian artists depicted Jesus and other figures as surrounded by coronas of light. The Vedic scriptures and teachings of the Rosicrucians, Tibetan and Indian Buddhists, as well as many Native American tribes describe the human energy field in detail. Even Pythagoras discussed the field, which he talked about as a luminous body. In fact, John White and Stanley Krippner, authors of *Future Science: Life Energies and the Physics of Paranormal Phenomena*, list 97 different cultures that reference the human aura, each describing the same phenomenon but calling it by a different name. Born in 1580, Belgian mystic, chemist, physiologist, and physician Jan Baptist van Helmont visualized the aura as a universal fluid that permeates everything.

The idea of fluidity and permeability being features of the aura has remained consistent throughout history. Franz

Mesmer, a German physician to whom we attribute the term *mesmerized*, suggested that both animate and inanimate objects were charged with a fluid, which he perceived as magnetic. This fluid, he believed, enabled material bodies to exert influence over each other, even at a distance. Baron Wilhelm von Reichenbach, a German chemist, also discovered several properties unique to the human energy field and determined that it shared similar properties to the electromagnetic field. Reichenbach also found that the human energy field related to different colors and that it could not only carry a charge but also flow around objects. He described the field on the left side of the body as a negative pole and the right side as a positive pole, similar to the ideas of Chinese medicine.

All these investigations have consistently revealed that the aura has a fluid or flowing state and that it is comprised of different colors, and therefore frequencies. It has also been consistently observed that the aura is permeable and penetrable and is magnetic in nature, although it also has electromagnetic properties. In early 1900s, it was discovered that the aura reacted to a person's state of mind and health. It was also observed that areas of congestion could be cleared to release negative mental and emotional patterns. In the 1930s, an English psychiatrist, Dr. Lawrence Bendit, together with his clairvoyant wife, Phoebe Bendit, observed the connection between the human energy field and health. Their observations were later mirrored and expanded by Dr. Dora Kunz, who spoke about every organ having its own field. That is, of course, also true for the overall subtle body, which has a specific frequency when healthy. When someone is ill, these frequencies alter. These disruption and related problems can be seen in the field. There are thousands upon thousands of intuitives across the planet who can see them. In fact, you can train yourself to see them too. Anybody can develop this ability with practice.

Dr. Zheng Rongliang of Lanzhou University in China used a unique biological detector to measure the flow of energy from a human body and showed that not only does the aura pulse but that not everyone's human energy field pulses at the same rate or intensity. This study was repeated by researchers at the Shanghai Atomic Nuclear Institute of Academia Sinica. Also, scientists from the Bioinformation Institute in Russia measured the biocurrents in the human biofield and discovered that people with a strong and widespread biofield can transfer energy more successfully. This research was later confirmed by the Medical Science Academy in Moscow. Another very interesting study by Dr. Valerie Hunt recorded the frequency of low-millivoltage signals emanating from the body during Rolfing sessions. When the wave patterns were analyzed, it was indeed discovered that the field consists of a number of different color bands, which correlate to the main chakras.

Barbara Ann Brennan summarizes all this scientific research to suggest that the auric field is made of *plasma*, possibly subatomic particles that move in clouds, which she refers to as the fifth state of matter. There is also another theory that the field is actually made of both electromagnetic radiation and an antimatter. This enables instant communication between energy fields of different people, as well as allows a shift of energy between this world and others. Even though we do not fully understand the mechanics of how exactly all this works, there is no question that it does. Some people still choose to poo-poo it, but the reality is if you do not consider the relationships between your biofield and your health, you will fall short. More often than not, those "mysterious" health problems people keep going in circles with have this energetic connection, which is why they cannot be resolved with biochemistry alone.

Balancing the Core Chakras

In this section, we will look more closely at the seven core chakras. We will look at how you can assess the health of your chakras and some strategies that can help you balance them.

There are many chakras, but I personally work with the main seven body chakras, as well the higher chakras. For our purposes, we will focus on the core seven, as their balance is critical from the point of view of our physical health. The energy flow through the chakras absolutely affects how we function on the mental, emotional, and physical level. Remember the Triangle of Healing we talked about at the very beginning? Everything affects everything else.

The mainstream seven chakra system is based on a Hindu chakra system that recognizes seven distinct *wheels* or *centers* of energy. Those wheels of energy along the human body's spinal column are in a state of constant flux, depending on the situations, people, and emotions that come into your life at any given time. This makes sense as we are talking about energy flow, which means constant movement. We already said that when we talk about energy, we are talking about constant vibration. Nothing rests. Each chakra possesses its own vibrational frequency, which is associated with a color. As you may already be aware, each of these energy centers corresponds to different aspects of our emotional and physical well-being due to their connection to organs and glands.

You can adjust your self-expression and health outcomes by becoming more aware of your energetic strengths and weaknesses at any given time and making sure your chakras are well-balanced. It is normal for your chakras to open and close depending on your personal circumstances so you should not really be micromanaging them. I suggest you check them regularly, e.g., once a week or when you feel you need to. As you work with chakras, over time you will intuitively know which ones may need extra attention to ensure optimal flow energy. So let us now look at each of the chakras and their connections to our emotional and physical health. I will also share my favorite strategies to optimize the functioning of your chakras.

Root Chakra (Muladhara)

Positioning: base of the spine
Color: red
Element: earth

The root chakra governs the functioning of the lower part of the body, including the lower spine and back, large intestine, and blood. Blockages may manifest as problems in any of those organs, e.g., back pain. This chakra governs confidence and survival instincts (fight-or-flight). It is connected to the basic needs and feelings of safety. If getting your basic needs met (e.g., having enough money for food or to pay bills, having stable housing, feeling safe in your home or in the world, etc.) is a constant struggle, chances are that your root chakra will benefit from healing work. When this chakra is blocked or imbalanced, this may manifest as feelings of insecurity, fear, aggressiveness, or low self-esteem. The person may be short-tempered, obsessive, paranoid, jealous, greedy, or restless and may suffer from eating disorders or addictions. Healing your root chakra empowers you to confidently face whatever life may bring you.

Root Chakra Questionnaire (the more questions you answer *yes* to, the more imbalance you have in this chakra)

1. *Do you often feel stuck and sluggish?*
2. *Do you feel stressed due to not being able to control external circumstances?*
3. *Do you have persistent financial problems?*
4. *Do you ever feel abandoned?*
5. *Do you feel disconnected from your body?*
6. *Do you feel insecure about life (i.e. do you feel like your basic needs in life are not being met or like you are constantly getting by or going without)?*
7. *Do you have any anger towards your body?*
8. *Do you feel you are not good enough the way you are?*
9. *Do you have any issues with your lower body parts (e.g., feet, knees, lower back, large bowel)?*

Balancing the Root Chakra
Affirmations:
- *I feel deeply rooted*
- *I am connected to my body*
- *I feel safe and secure in my body*
- *I have what I need*

Words (mantras) that you can repeat over and over: *I am safe, supported, secure, calm, grounded*

Essential oils: patchouli, sandalwood, myrrh, vetiver

Examples of yoga poses:
- sitting cross legged combined with deep, slow breathing
- warriors
- Hindi squat

Gemstones: jasper, bloodstone, red carnelian, garnet, hematite, smokey quartz

Sound: 396 Hz Solfeggio frequency

Sacral Chakra (Swadhisthana)

Positioning: just below the navel
Color: orange
Element: water

The sacral chakra is associated primarily with emotional regulation. It is often referred to as the seat of our emotions. It is also associated with the sense of taste and with reproductive function. Physical manifestations of this chakra not working properly include: sex hormone imbalances, infertility, ectopic pregnancies, miscarriages, endometriosis, ovarian cysts, abdominal cramps, and urinary infections. Because of its positioning, this chakra is also associated with pleasure, whether sensual or related to your daily life experiences. Both emotional overactivity and emotional disconnect are signs of an imbalance. Other signs include: excessive neediness, codependency, indulgence, poor boundaries, fear of happiness or pleasure, self-sabotage, lack of creativity or authenticity, low or overly high libido, pessimism, depression, rigidity, envy, jealousy, anger, and rage. A common symptom of the sacral chakra imbalance is also a tendency to get consumed in fantasies about life's pleasures instead of actually enjoying them.

A balanced sacral chakra enables us to creatively deal with what emerges from our experience, live as our authentic selves without fear, and develop appropriate responses governed by our emotional intelligence. It also allows us to fully experience intimacy and love without being judgmental about our desires.

Sacral Chakra Questionnaire

1. *Do you have difficulty with intimacy?*
2. *Do you believe that sex is bad or that it can hurt you?*
3. *Do you believe you have to be sexy to be loved?*
4. *Have you ever suffered sexual abuse?*
5. *Do you often feel hurt and/or confused?*
6. *Do you tend to get overly emotional, or do you feel disconnected from your emotions and struggle to feel them?*
7. *Do you struggle with your self-image?*
8. *Do you have tendency to end up in unsuccessful/toxic relationships?*
9. *Do you have difficulties setting healthy boundaries?*
10. *Do you have any physical issues relating to your reproductive or urinary organs?*

Balancing the Sacral Chakra
Affirmations:

- *I have healthy emotional responses*
- *I have healthy boundaries*
- *I love and enjoy my body*
- *I know how to take care of my emotional needs*

Words that you can repeat over and over: *I am receptive, flexible, adaptable, creative, emotionally connected.*

Essential oils: ylang ylang, sandalwood, sweet orange, neroli, jasmine, clary sage

Examples of yoga poses:

- butterfly pose
- half happy baby (dead bug)
- extended swan pose

Gemstones: carnelian, tiger's eye, orange calcite, orange moonstone, sunstone

Sound: 417 Hz Solfeggio frequency

Solar Plexus Chakra (Manipura)

Positioning: stomach area
Color: yellow
Element: fire

This is a center of your personal power. When well balanced, this chakra enables you to have control over your thoughts and emotional responses, set healthy boundaries, and be at peace with yourself. At the physical level, this chakra is associated with digestive function but also the skin and immunity. Any issues with digestion or dysfunction of any of the digestive organs indicate an imbalance. Symptoms associated with excessive energy in the solar plexus chakra include being: controlling, dominant, overindulgent, intolerant, overly critical, perfectionistic, constantly on the go (a human doing rather than a human being), and being excessively competitive. Symptoms of deficiency in this chakra include: insecurity, victimhood, anxiety, fear, poor appetite, passivity, lack of confidence, low self-esteem, poor self-image, inability to focus, lack of organization, and weak will. Any time you feel disempowered for whatever reason, this chakra is being negatively affected.

Solar Plexus Chakra Questionnaire

1. *Do you often feel powerless or victimized?*
2. *Do you handle criticism or rejection badly?*
3. *Do you feel like you have to achieve all the time?*
4. *Do you have perfectionistic tendencies?*
5. *Do you ever give your power away to others to keep peace in relationships?*
6. *Do you have difficulties pursuing your dreams due to low self-esteem?*
7. *Do you have poor self-image? Do you dislike your body?*
8. *Do you have any physical issues related to your stomach, liver, pancreas, gall*
9. *bladder, intestines, intestines, or spleen?*

Balancing the Solar Plexus Chakra
Affirmations:

- *I love and accept myself*
- *I am happy being me*
- *I feel empowered to live authentically*
- *I am at peace with myself*

Words that you can repeat over and over: *I am worthy, powerful, strong, confident*

Essential oils: chamomile, lavender, rosemary, ginger, peppermint, lemon, juniper

Yoga poses:

- seated twist
- lunge twist
- child's pose twist
- intense pose twist

Gemstones: citrine, lemon quartz, yellow jasper, pyrite, tiger's eye, amber (resin)

Sound: 528 Hz Solfeggio frequency

Heart Chakra (Anahata)

Positioning: center of the chest
Color: green
Element: air

The heart chakra is associated with love—not just towards others but also self-love. On the physical level, this chakra is connected to the physical heart and also the lungs. When the heart chakra is deficient or closed, it may translate into: being withdrawn, avoiding social interactions, being overly critical of others and oneself, lacking empathy, and feeling isolated. On the other hand, if the heart chakra is overly open, it may manifest as: being overly demanding of others, being clingy, trying to fulfill other people's perceived needs to one's own detriment, feeling like a victim, and losing a sense of personal boundaries.

Healing the heart chakra is felt as a boost in energy, positivity, love, compassion, and increased sense of connectedness to life. The heart chakra is super important not just because it is associated with love but also because it is the chakra that connects the bottom three chakras with the top three chakras. Stress or imbalance in neighboring chakras often influences the state of the heart chakra. It is important to realize that as humanity is progressing in its ascension process, the heart chakra will become much more dominant. This is because the new era we are moving into is going to be driven by love and compassion. This is an additional reason why it is recommended to pay more attention to this chakra and to keep it open and balanced.

Heart Chakra Questionnaire

1. *Do you have trust issues?*
2. *Do you feel like you have to please others to earn their approval/affection?*
3. *Have you been hurt in the past and now feel like you have to guard yourself?*
4. *Do you struggle with giving and receiving love and being compassionate?*
5. *Do you struggle to let go of grudges? Do you difficulties forgiving?*
6. *Do you get jealous?*
7. *Do you feel like your life lacks love and/or joy?*
8. *Do you have physical imbalances, such as: asthma, heart disease, lung disease, breast issues, lymphatic congestion, or middle back problems?*

Balancing the Heart Chakra
Affirmations:

- *I am open to love*
- *I deeply and completely love and accept myself*
- *I forgive myself and others*
- *I feel connected to other living beings*

Words to be repeated over and over: *I am loving, connected, compassionate, free*

Essential oils: helichrysum, lemon (self-love), bergamot, jasmine, lavender, sweet marjoram

Examples of yoga poses:
- bow pose
- cobra or baby cobra
- camel pose

Gemstones: green jasper, jade, green tourmaline, green aventurine, emerald, rose quartz

Sound: 639 Hz Solfeggio frequency

Throat Chakra (Vishuddha)

Positioning: base of the throat
Color: blue
Element: ether

This energy center is associated with communication, creativity, and self-expression. The throat chakra controls the thyroid gland and the endocrine system. That means it is responsible for the regulation and flow of hormones and the function of the trachea, mouth, esophagus, teeth, nose, ears, and carotid arteries. Manifestations such as hoarseness, laryngitis, thyroid issues, speech impairments, and tinnitus are associated with the throat chakra imbalance. A blockage can also initiate behaviors indicating insecurity and a lack of control, such as: being manipulative, lying, arrogance, anxiety, fear, diminished self-esteem, and compulsive or excessive eating. A deficiency is characteristic of people who are quiet, shy, in fear of speaking out, or secretive, whereas an overactive throat chakra will be characterized by excessive talking, poor listening, or speaking loudly.

Throat Chakra Questionnaire
1. *Do you have difficulties expressing what you feel think?*

2. *Do you feel inclined to go along with others so you don't upset anyone? Do you have problems with being your authentic self? Do you hold that back?*

3. *Are you frustrated because you don't feel that other people hear what you have to say?*

4. *Do you feel creativity is not your thing?*

5. *Do you have physical imbalances that include: thyroid issues, sore throats, laryngitis, TMJ, ear infections, any facial problems (chin, cheek, lips, tongue problems), or neck and shoulder pain?*

Balancing the Throat Chakra
Affirmations:
- *I feel good about speaking my truth*
- *I communicate my feelings with ease*
- *I value integrity and honesty*
- *I choose to express gratitude for what I have*

Words to be repeated: *I am honest, truthful, authentic, creative*

Essential oils: frankincense, geranium, peppermint, eucalyptus, roman and German chamomile, lavender

Examples of yoga poses:
- cow and cat (open the throat)
- fish pose
- neck stretches and neck rotation

Gemstones: turquoise, blue aquamarine, blue sodalite, lapis lazuli, azurite

Sound: 741 Hz Solfeggio frequency

Third Eye Chakra (Ajna)

Positioning: forehead
Color: indigo
Element: light

This energy center governs the pineal gland and your vision, intuition, memory, and imagination. The idea behind awakening the third eye, or brow chakra, is to see things more clearly within and outside of the physical realm. An open third eye chakra makes you very intuitive and enables you to see things as they truly are. This chakra works in partnership with the crown chakra to complete the chakra "circuit" and help you reach new levels of awareness. When this chakra is overactive, the mind can go into overdrive, much like it would if you had a few cups of coffee. This can make it difficult to concentrate and can produce overwhelm, obsessive, intrusive thoughts or memories, and in some cases, hallucinations. On the other end, an energy deficiency can also hinder your ability to focus and affect your ability to process and remember information. It can also make you indecisive, procrastinate, become fearful of the unknown, and crumble under pressure. Additional issues that can arise from a blocked or imbalanced third eye chakra include: insomnia, high blood pressure, depression, anxiety, headaches, and migraines.

Third Eye Chakra Questionnaire

1. *Do you struggle to find meaning in life and often ask yourself: why am I here?*
2. *Do you feel disconnected from your intuition? Do you struggle to trust your inner guidance?*
3. *Do you have difficulties making decisions?*

4. *Are you feeling lost when it comes to your spiritual purpose and path in life?*

5. *Do you feel that there is something wrong or out of alignment?*

6. *Do you often feel moody or volatile?*

7. *Do you daydream often?*

8. *Do you have an inability to learn from other people's mistakes?*

9. *Do you have physical imbalances that include: headaches, blurred vision, sinus issues, eyestrain, seizures, hearing loss, or hormone function?*

Balancing the Third Eye Chakra
Affirmations:
- *I am in touch with my inner guidance*
- *I listen to my deepest wisdom*
- *I seek to understand and to learn from my life experiences*
- *I trust my intuition*

Words to be repeated: *I am intuitive, trusting, connected* (to my higher self, the universe)

Essential oils: bay laurel, jasmine, melissa, neroli, clary sage, German chamomile, sandalwood

Example of yoga poses:
- down dog (connecting the body and the mind)
- one legged dog with bringing your knee to the third eye
- flat back extend focusing your third eye forward
- child's pose (pressing your third eye into the floor)

Gemstones: lapis lazuli, sodalite, iolite, tanzanite

Sound: 852 Hz Solfeggio frequency

Crown Chakra (Sahasrara)

Positioning: top of the head
Color: violet or white
Element: space

This chakra is represented by a lotus flower with a thousand petals. This chakra is what allows us to move beyond individual materialistic needs and connect with the universe as a whole. Opening the crown chakra brings you spiritual insight and the ability to live with confidence in all aspects of life. An unbalanced crown chakra can play a role in learning disabilities, sleep disorders, mental illness, and comas. A deficiency in the crown chakra is characterized by greed, materialism, cynicism, closed mindedness, and being a know-it-all. It tends to cause subtle, systemic problems, such as: brain fog (inability to think clearly), chronic fatigue, depression, migraines, and headaches. On the other hand, an overactive crown chakra may be an issue if somebody experiences hypersensitivity to light and sound, as well as neurological or endocrine disorders. Excess energy in this chakra can also be associated with boredom, frustration, a sense of elitism, obsessive attachment to spirituality, living in fantasy and lacking connection to self and reality, and spiritual bypass.

Crown Chakra Questionnaire

1. *Do you feel lonely, insignificant or aimless?*
2. *Do you have a strong attachment to material possessions and achievements (and define yourself according to them) and are disconnected from the spiritual side of life?*
3. *Do you feel a lack of connection or guidance from a higher power? Do you feel disconnected from the source/universe/*

divine? Do not believe you are part of something greater than yourself?

4. *Do you feel unworthy of spiritual help or angry that the higher power has abandoned you?*
5. *Do you tend to over-analyze everything?*
6. *Do you use spirituality to avoid dealing with your emotions or with life?*
7. *Are you hypersensitive to light and sound?*
8. *Do you suffer from migraines and tension headaches?*
9. *Do you suffer from physical imbalances that include: depression, sensitivity to light, sound, environment?*

Balancing the Crown Chakra
Affirmations:
- *I seek experiences that nourish my spirit*
- *I am connected with the wisdom of the universe*
- *I am at peace*
- *I am part of the Divine*

Words to be repeated: *I am whole, conscious, connected, peaceful*

Essential oils: jasmine, rose and lavender, sandalwood, frankincense, myrrh, benzoin, helichrysum

Example of yoga poses:
- in a seated position take deep slow breaths to be fully present with your hands in a prayer position on the top of your head
- sun salutations
- body circles

Gemstones: amethyst, clear quarz, sugilite, spirit quartz, howlite, selenite

Sound: 963 Hz Solfeggio frequency

In addition, you can access my meditation to balance your energy field and your chakras in the Additional Resources. I hope you enjoy it!

Frequencies of Emotions

We have said many times already that emotions are energy in motion. Emotions have frequencies, and these frequencies have been measured. Take a closer look at the diagram. At the bottom, measured in hertz (Hz), we have shame at only 20 hertz. That means shame is a very dense, very low vibration emotional state. Do you remember when I said that shame is one of the heaviest emotions, as it is connected to self-loathing and eroded identity? You can see that here. On the other end of the spectrum is enlightenment and peace at 700 – 1000 Hz. This is exactly why we say that internal harmony heals.

If you consistently emit frequencies this high, you will be healthy because disease is associated with low, dense vibrations. This means disease cannot exist in the body if you consistently emit such high frequencies. I hope you can see that. However, most people have a lot of unhealthy guilt and shame, as well as chronic fear and anger. They are at this getting-by level. This is another reason why neutralizing these chronic toxic emotional states is very important while at the same time working towards peace and enlightenment by cultivating self-love, love and compassion towards others, and joy. At the very least, people who want to be relatively healthy should aim to be in acceptance most of the time. All the work you are doing on trauma, self-worth, beliefs, and your biofield is helping you ascend along this spectrum.

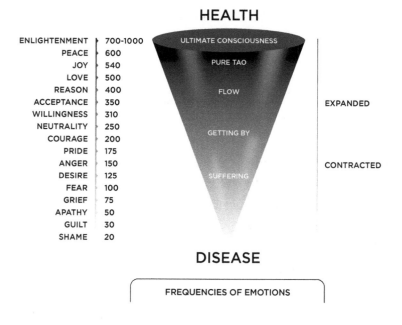

HEALTH

ENLIGHTENMENT	700-1000	ULTIMATE CONSCIOUSNESS
PEACE	600	
JOY	540	PURE TAO
LOVE	500	
REASON	400	FLOW
ACCEPTANCE	350	
WILLINGNESS	310	EXPANDED
NEUTRALITY	250	
COURAGE	200	GETTING BY
PRIDE	175	
ANGER	150	CONTRACTED
DESIRE	125	
FEAR	100	SUFFERING
GRIEF	75	
APATHY	50	
GUILT	30	
SHAME	20	

DISEASE

FREQUENCIES OF EMOTIONS

Setting Energetic Boundaries & Healing Ancestral Trauma

Before we proceed to assessing your levels of energetic sensitivity and looking at how you can set energetic boundaries to protect your energetic field, I want to emphasize that this work has NOTHING to do with religion. There is much scientific merit to doing biofield work. I shared some research highlights, but there is much more if you want to delve deeper. You definitely do not have to be religious to do this work, and you do not even have to be spiritual. I know agnostics who utilize these tools because they connect with the science of it. That said, in my opinion, you cannot really reach optimal levels of health if you are not prepared to entertain that you are part of something bigger than yourself.

For one, people who only believe in the 3D physical world and nothing else tend to be fearful of many things (e.g., fear of the unknown, fear of death, fear of losing their material possessions, etc.). Having all that fear is emotionally toxic, which is far from promoting an optimal mindset, and therefore health. On the other hand, if you do believe that you are part of something greater than yourself, you are prepared to look at life from the point of view of energy and consciousness, not just your immediate 3D reality. Appreciating the interconnectedness of everything in the universe already makes you spiritual, even if you may not think of yourself in that way. This is important because spirituality plays a big role in health and healing.

So let us now look at assessing the level of your energetic sensitivity. First of all, generally, most people dealing with chronic health issues will have a degree of energetic sensitivity. You may have heard of this being described as being an empath. When you think about it, this is quite logical because in those first years of our lives, we are dealing with so much as children. People around us have to be pretty switched on to satisfy our needs properly, which is why so many people end up with those attachment adaptations we have discussed previously. If we now throw increased sensitivity into the mix, that creates even more potential for that child to be traumatized. It is particularly unfortunate when a sensitive child has narcissistic parent or parents. That is a bad combo. If a child has a parent who is a narcissist, then they will always be trying to win the love and approval of the parent who is not capable of unconditional love. It is always about making the parent look good by being a good little girl or boy.

In addition, in our toxic Western culture, children are often told not to be so sensitive and are expected to just get on with it. I would say 8 to 9 out of 10 people I have worked with over the years have been empaths. This is obviously a spectrum. You can be more or less sensitive. It is definitely not the same for everyone, but one thing I have observed is that there is a correlation between the degree of sensitivity and the severity of somebody's illness. By illness severity I mean number of symptoms, how long somebody has been sick, and how serious the illness is.

We are going to go through some questions in a moment to assess where you are on the empath spectrum. Many people in professions where you care for others (e.g., nurses, therapists, social workers) are empaths. The more of an empath you are, the more you need to be disciplined about your energy hygiene, as well setting really solid boundaries. We have covered toxic traits previously. As an empath, you need to be particularly aware of toxic people in your environment, as they will drain your energy greatly if you let them. I am not just talking here about narcissists and sociopaths. You also have to be aware of those *poor me* type people who are stuck in victimhood.

Energetic Sensitivity Assessment

The more statements are true for you, the more of an empath you are and the more it is important for you to protect your energy field and shield yourself.

1. You are highly sensitive to loud noises, bright lights chemicals, and/or odors.

2. You have a strong desire to fix people and relieve their stress and/or you love to take care of people and put their needs ahead of your own.

3. You tend to avoid social situations or crowded places because they drain you.

4. You experience sudden mood shifts; you feel fine for a while and then can suddenly feel anxious or low for no apparent reason.

5. You tend to get overwhelmed a lot.

6. You love to spend time alone and need to recharge after being around other people or in a crowd.

7. Too much togetherness in a relationship or friendship can feel suffocating and anxiety provoking.

8. You are spiritual but feel like you are still searching for your purpose.

9. You often choose activities that are quiet (tend to socially isolate).

10. You find yourself attracting energy vampires, narcissists, or toxic relationships repeatedly.

11. You allow other people to take advantage of your kindness.

12. You have been described by others as "overly sensitive," shy, or introverted.

13. Arguments or yelling make you feel ill.

14. You feel like you do not fit in.

15. You prefer one-to-one interactions or small groups rather than large gatherings.

16. You often overeat to cope with stress.

17. You startle easily.

18. You react strongly to caffeine and/or medications.

19. You have a low pain threshold.

20. You often forget to include self-care in your daily life.

21. You absorb other people's stress, emotions, or symptoms.

22. You feel overwhelmed by multitasking and prefer doing one thing at a time.

23. You find nature regenerating.

24. You need a long time to recuperate after being with difficult people or energy vampires.

25. You feel better in small cities or the country than large cities.

Now that you know where you are on the empath spectrum, I will share with you some simple strategies that will help you protect your energy field. Just remember that being an empath is different from being empathetic. Being empathetic is when you care about other people and you do not want to see them harmed. Being an empath is different. You can actually feel another person's emotions, happiness, fear, anger, sadness in your own body. In empaths, the brain's mirror neuron system, a specialized group of cells that are responsible for compassion, is thought to be particularly active. As a result, empaths can absorb other people's energies (both positive and negative) into their own bodies. Also, how empaths process dopamine, the pleasure hormone, is a bit different. They do not need a big surge of dopamine that extroverts tend to need. At times, it may even be difficult to tell if you are feeling your own emotions or somebody else's. The more you build your self-awareness and the more you get to know yourself at a really deep level, the easier it becomes to tell what is yours and what is not.

Being an empath has incredible benefits, such as enhanced intuition, more compassion, creativity, and a deeper connection to other people. However, if you do not balance your energies and protect yourself, this state of high sensitivity can leave you exhausted, overwhelmed, overstimulated, stressed, and negative. When unmanaged, energetic hypersensitivity overstimulates the nervous system, which, over time, will contribute to mental and physical health issues. Empaths who are not aware of any of this often use food, alcohol, and drugs to numb their emotions and make things more bearable for themselves. That is, of course, not only unnecessary but also damaging. There are better ways to navigate energetic sensitivity.

Protecting Your Energy Field

We can protect our field in a variety of different ways. I have already shared my energy balancing meditation with you. Here are some other strategies you can use.

Protective Gemstones

Some of the best gemstones that can protect us from negative energy include: black tourmaline, obsidian, black onyx, shungite, clear quartz, smokey quartz, diamond, amber (resin), hematite, jet, amethyst, labradorite, malachite, and rainbow moonstone. There are others. You can use these as jewelry or carry a stone in your pocket. You can also have them as orgonites and place them on your desk or place a stone on your desk if you work in an office. One point I would like to make about using gemstones is that most gemstones need to be periodically cleared and charged, so you need to be aware of that. I recommend that you look up how to do that and which gemstones require it.

Salt

Having a salts bath is very effective for clearing your energy field. You can also sprinkle some sea salt around your desk at work or around your home. You need to leave it for a few hours before cleaning it up.

Smudging

Smudging is an ancient practice or ritual where you burn dried sage or other dried herbs to cleanse a person or area. You can use sage, sandalwood, mugwort, or palo santo for this purpose.

Mudras

Mudras are hand gestures that carry specific goals of channeling your body's energy flow.

Mudra of Earth (Prithvi Mudra) is a mudra of protection.

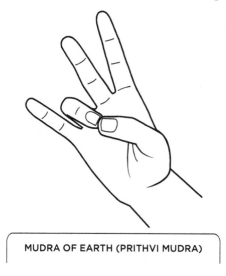

MUDRA OF EARTH (PRITHVI MUDRA)

Kashyapa Mudra is also a powerful protection mudra. You can use it anytime you face toxic people, energy vampires, or people with bad attitudes.

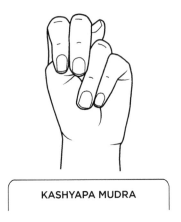

KASHYAPA MUDRA

Energetic Boundary Work

1. Energetic Cord Cutting

We have used this visualization previously when doing forgiveness work, but you can also use it to remove any energetic connections that do not serve you. Just remember to cut all the cords and put yourself and the other person in two separate protective bubbles. Wish them well and imagine them drifting away into the distance until they disappear out of sight.

2. Ring of Fire

This is a great visualization to help you clear any energetic influences or negativity you do not want in your energy field. Close your eyes and take a few deep cleansing breaths. Be in your own body and imagine a ring of fire around you burning off and transmuting anything you want to get rid of energetically. Focus on the energy being cleansed and purified by the fire for a couple of minutes.

3. Shielding

Whenever you are dealing with people who drain your energy, imagine you are holding a shield in front of you. This can be a very simple shield that protects your chest and stomach area or a full-body shield. Choose what you want it to look like and what it is made of. You can imagine it in an instant with an intention to repel any energy that is not good for you. If you are a sensitive person, I recommend you do that when you deal with crowds as well (e.g., going into a crowded supermarket or traveling on public transportation). You can also imagine yourself in a mirror ball with the reflective surface on the outside. Use whatever resonates with you most.

Healing Ancestral Trauma

In this section, I want to talk about ancestral trauma and how you can do some of this work yourself. At some point, you might decide to work with a psychic healer who specializes in this type of work, but you can definitely do some of this work yourself. In fact, simple visualizations are often sufficient. Some people want to overcomplicate this work. My experience shows that in most cases that is not necessary. However, at times, professional help might be needed.

The reason why I did not start this book with healing ancestral trauma is because I do not want to encourage the mindset of *I am feeling X, but it must be somebody else's*. The reality is that most of people's emotional layers are created by them internally, so first you want to recognize and heal those. If somebody watches mainstream news every day, that is a lifestyle choice. They then become fearful and anxious, which leads them to self-sabotage, or getting sick, or placing limitations on what they can achieve. Let me be clear: that has nothing to do with their ancestors. We need to take responsibility for our choices and focus on healing what we have created ourselves.

However, there are patterns that we have inherited from our ancestors. Those can be perpetuated if we are running them without any self-awareness. When somebody has those repetitive destructive patterns (e.g., attracting narcissists in relationships or making money and then losing everything over and over), this usually means there is an element of influence from previous generations. While some people jump into ancestral trauma first, which I think is inadvisable, other people deny that there is any connection between what they are going through and what they ancestors may have experienced. That is also a mistake. You know you are influenced by something that goes however many generations back if you have addressed your limiting beliefs, healed your traumas and your inner child, and there is still something hanging over you. It is possible that your inner child may need more healing, but when you really have done the work thoroughly and your emotional or physical symptoms are still not clearing, then you absolutely need to look deeper into ancestral work. Also, sometimes people can have phobias, or even PTSD, which cannot be explained by anything that they experienced themselves.

If you have identified yourself as an empath, you already know that you can pick up other people's energy easily. Even if you are not high on the energetic sensitivity scale, you are unequivocally affected by other people's energy, as well as the energy of places. It is important to recognize that even though the more you do this work, the more easily you can recognize what is energetically yours and what is not, it is not black and white. Ancestral trauma can be experienced concurrently with personal issues as you are healing them or independently of them, meaning these issues can be intertwined and often it is difficult to tell what is what. This is because those ancestral traumas tend to relate to our own lives while simultaneously being very ancient in origin. So you may have certain patterns precisely because your ancestors had certain traumas. But again, if you strip those other layers that we have covered so far, you will be clearer on what else needs to be addressed. In some cases, if you thoroughly address the aspects covered so far in the book, you will not need to do any specific ancestral healing work, but often this type of healing is necessary to complete the process.

When you are thinking about your ancestors, back to the times when people had to be on the lookout for real threats, those who were paranoid and jumpy had more of a chance of surviving than those who were happy and not as alert to actual threats, such as wild animals. From the point of view of nervous system development, we already said that this is where our fight, flight, and freeze responses comes from. That paranoid ancestor who survived passed that survival mechanism on to the next generation and the next. So now we are here with this incredibly fine-tuned survival mechanism. This is also why we have a negativity bias. It all comes from our ancestors, who had to learn how to survive. But now we are learning that this mechanism can be altered. It can be relaxed. We can make our nervous system less reactive and we can remodel our brain, which you have been doing by engaging with all the techniques I am sharing with you. Your ancestral fear is connected to your cells and body. This is why I said from the beginning that dropping into the body is critical to healing. So, as you can see, you have already been working through your intergenerational and ancestral baggage by doing all this work so far. What is interesting is that when you do this work on yourself, you are also automatically healing your ancestors. In addition, because we are talking about the quantum field, you are also healing your family line into the future.

Just like with beliefs, when looking at your ancestry and your family's past, which you may or may not know, you need to decide what is serving you that you want to keep and what is not serving you that you want to let go of. Some people choose to do some research into their family history, but you do not have to do that. Essentially, you will feel it in your body. When it comes to intergenerational and ancestral trauma, you absolutely have the power to make sure that certain patterns stop with you. If you resolve them, you will not pass them on. So you need to reflect a bit, if you have not already, on what patterns have run in your family. Consider that events have occurred in yours and other people's families that have caused you and other people in your life to think and act in certain ways. Rather than blame, approach it with curiosity and compassion and ask questions such as:

What happened in my partner's family that he or she is acting this way or getting triggered in this way?

What is happening between my partner and me, and in our energy field, that is producing this behavior in my child or my animal? What is being mirrored? What needs to be healed?

There are some key things to keep in mind about ancestral clearing and how to do it:

1. Intention is everything.

A simple intention to want to break the cycle is going to positively impact your neurology. It has been shown that when you say *no* to something, it can take as little as 12 seconds to establish a new neural connection. Twelve seconds! If you are consistently doing it, your old pathways start to break down within three weeks. This is why I am recommending you do those mediations I am offering continuously for several weeks before you move to the maintenance phase. We do not need to know what trauma, events, or patterns we are clearing with regards our ancestors and what they experienced. You certainly do not need to know every last detail about them. That is not that important. This is energetic work. We just have to want to clear those traumas and patterns.

2. This work is about reconnecting to the innate divine intelligence that guides us in every area of our lives.

Again, somebody who is not at all spiritual and omits this part of psycho-energetic healing may find that this is exactly what may be holding them back. If so, they will be unable to progress. This is one reason why spirituality is important to achieve deeper healing.

3. This work is about asking and releasing.

As I said before, you do not need to overcomplicate this process. You can simply request that Source (in whatever form this appears to you), or the universe, helps you let go of whatever you are trying to release. Ask to be assisted in clearing whatever it was that contributed to your situation that has been causing you pain, discomfort, or disease. Sometimes it is really that simple, provided you are prepared to surrender, trust, and let go.

4. Emphasize the highest good.

Ensure that you ask Source to allow ancestral clearing to take place for the highest good of everyone affected.

5. Do not overanalyze this.

This is a heart-driven process, so resist being analytical about it. To facilitate this process of clearing you need to get out of your head, drop into the body, and connect with your heart.

Ancestral Healing Visualizations

First of all, remember the energetic cord cutting technique if there is anybody on your mother's or father's side of the family that you specifically want to be energetically free from.

This next visualization for ancestral healing is designed to help you connect more deeply with your loving ancestors and help support those ancestors who need healing. You can read it first and then go through the process with your eyes closed. It does not need to be exact. Your mind will take you where you need to go. This is just a guide to give you an idea of what we are trying to achieve. You can then adjust it to suit you and fill in the details.

Make yourself comfortable, close your eyes, feel your body, and feel connected to the ground. Open up your heart space by bringing your shoulder blades closer together. Adjust your chin if necessary so there is a good flow of energy through your throat chakra. Relax your jaw and relax the tongue inside your mouth. Connect with your breath. Low belly breathing, slow inhales, even slower exhales. With every exhalation, you release and let go. Now recall your energy from any place you may have left some of it this week or last week. Allow your energy and only your energy to come back to you right here and now. With every inhale you allow yourself to be present, and with every exhale you let go a little bit more. Imagine yourself in a beautiful, peaceful, safe place in nature. Wherever it is, know that it is right for you. Feel connected to Mother Earth. Take in colors, textures, and sounds of that place, relaxing more and more deeply. Now look around and find yourself a spot to sit or lie down. Make yourself comfortable. Now imagine a golden sphere of light that represents all of your deepest knowing. Imagine this light filling your crown chakra and then your entire body. You know that you are already in a process of healing, releasing limiting beliefs, issues, attachments, traumas, ancestral patterns, past lives and anything else that is not serving you. You are healing right now, and forgiveness is getting easier and easier for you every day. With every breath in, you are expanding your heart space and you are expanding into forgiveness, which is the greatest way to free ourselves and allow ourselves to move forward. As the light travels further down your body and fills your root chakra, you know it is safe for you to connect with your ancestors. Imagine from your feet you have roots extending into the Earth, like a beautiful tree connecting with your ancestors. Now allow the light to fill the space around you, this egg-shaped space that is your field. Allow the light to fill your field, feeling calm and protected. As you are relaxing in your place in nature, grounded and protected, imagine your loving ancestors emerging and coming forward toward you, full of happiness and love. As you breathe in, you allow yourself to absorb their positive energy, their love and joy. Your beloved ancestors are forming a circle around you and they are showering you with positive energy, healing, love, and gratitude. They know that as you are working on yourself and you are releasing your limiting beliefs, your traumas, you are healing your ancestral lineages as well. In that moment, you feel connected and you feel that they are always there supporting you and that you can always return to this place to connect with them. Now see the sphere of golden light within the circle that your ancestors have formed, and if there is a pattern that you are aware of, that is not serving you, that you are in the process of clearing, place this pattern in the center of the sphere of light so that it can be released and healed now. Now imagine your beloved ancestors in the circle calling on any ancestors who need healing to also come to the center of the healing light. You now see some ancestors come forward to be healed, for their patterns to be released. They may have started some of the patterns that you want to release as a result of their traumas, indoctrination, or whatever else, but the important thing is that they are now coming forward and stepping into the light to have their patterns released and healed. Maybe that pattern helped them to survive but it no longer serves and is now being healed, released, and transformed. Take a few deeper breaths, now focusing on assisting with that release. You rest in knowing that your loving ancestors will continue to support you. They will also support those ancestors who need healing until those unhelpful patterns are fully released and transformed. Thank your loving ancestors for their support. Thank them for supporting and holding you. Now you see them waving goodbye, knowing you can always return to this place and meet them again. You feel good and appreciative. As you return back to your conscious awareness, make sure you can feel your body by wriggling you fingers and your toes. Connect back to your breath and open your eyes.

Hopefully, you were able to connect with this method of ancestral healing. There are many methods, of course. Some people like the idea of having a little altar in their house, some space dedicated to their ancestors, where they may have candles, crystals, or whatever else. If you decide to do this, just don't have it in your bedroom because this can be powerful energy you are dealing with, and you do not want your ancestors keeping you up at night!

Dealing with Ascension Symptoms & Optimizing Energy Flow in Your Spaces

In order to keep your energy field balanced and healthy, you need to also consider the ascension process, geopathic stress, and man-made electromagnetic fields. You may be aware that the Earth and humanity as a whole are currently going through a process of ascension, which in this context simply means evolution of consciousness. This process has been going on for some years now, but many people started to be much more aware of it since the start of 2020. This is reflected in the Schumann resonance increasing ever higher. Winfred Schumann, in the early 1960s, was the first scientist who accurately measured the electromagnetic frequencies of the Earth's atmosphere, or Schumann resonances. Our bodies, our brains, our DNA are calibrated to and dependent on the Earth's frequencies. There is a direct relationship between these frequencies and our brain wave activity.

The process of ascension is about aligning with your higher self and with Source. Awakening and spirituality are part of this ascension. As you learn to take control of your awareness, you are able to "wake up" to the authentic nature of your spirit and to empower yourself to consciously align with higher consciousness in every moment. There are many ascension teachers out there who are helping people navigate this journey, so if you want to know more about it, you can follow them. The reason I am mentioning it here is because through this process more and more light is coming into your body and your overall vibrational frequency is increasing. This is obviously a great thing, but as your body is changing, you may experience certain symptoms, so I want you to be aware of those and what to do. Be aware that this process is not something you can opt out of. It is a done deal. Sooner or later, everybody remaining on the Earth plane will embody higher frequencies of love, compassion, happiness, kindness, freedom, peace, and sovereignty. What is not going to have the right to exist as we ascend to those higher levels of consciousness is greed, manipulation, control, fear, or any other dense states.

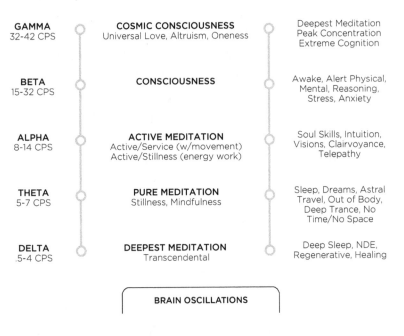

GAMMA 32-42 CPS	**COSMIC CONSCIOUSNESS** Universal Love, Altruism, Oneness	Deepest Meditation Peak Concentration Extreme Cognition
BETA 15-32 CPS	**CONSCIOUSNESS**	Awake, Alert Physical, Mental, Reasoning, Stress, Anxiety
ALPHA 8-14 CPS	**ACTIVE MEDITATION** Active/Service (w/movement) Active/Stillness (energy work)	Soul Skills, Intuition, Visions, Clairvoyance, Telepathy
THETA 5-7 CPS	**PURE MEDITATION** Stillness, Mindfulness	Sleep, Dreams, Astral Travel, Out of Body, Deep Trance, No Time/No Space
DELTA .5-4 CPS	**DEEPEST MEDITATION** Transcendental	Deep Sleep, NDE, Regenerative, Healing

BRAIN OSCILLATIONS

The bottom line is that these massive shifts in the Earth's frequencies, which ultimately are a wonderful thing because they are taking us towards a much better world and reality, can cause us to experience certain symptoms as the body is trying to adjust. Some common symptoms include: difficulty sleeping or waking up, attention deficit or lack of focus, memory issues (especially short-term), lack of drive or enthusiasm, physical sensations (e.g., humming or vibrating inside your body), increased fear and anxiety, difficulty breathing, agitation, feeling easily irritated or provoked, digestive issues or discomfort, skin issues (dryness, eruptions), muscle spasms or random twitching, vibrations in your extremities, headaches, fatigue, electrical zaps, tooth pain, ringing in the ears, sensitivity to light and sounds, all-over body ache, or swinging from one symptom to its opposite for no apparent reason.

These symptoms can have other root causes, obviously. I am not suggesting if you have any of these symptoms that you assume they are related to the ascension process, but if they are a reasonably recent thing, or they turn up out of nowhere, or they come and go, this may be related to the ascension, so just keep that in mind. All these mental and physical symptoms are about purging what no longer serves us. We are doing this on the individual and collective level. Other collective symptoms of the ascension are instability, chaos, and polarization. For now do your best to navigate that and look forward to everything getting rebalanced as we are ascending and moving towards stability and unity.

Strategies for Dealing with Ascension Symptoms

So what do you do if the ascension process is jarring on your system? The best thing to do is to keep yourself grounded as much as possible. In this context, to be *grounded*, or *grounding yourself*, essentially means staying connected to the present moment without being hijacked by your thoughts, emotions, or whatever is happening in the external. There are many ways to keep yourself grounded:

- visualize your feet are roots of a tree and you are connecting your roots to the Earth
- focus on your inhales and exhales (deep, slow breathing is best for grounding)
- practice qigong, yoga, tai chi, or engage in other activities, such as walking or dancing
- do meditations that bring you into the body, such as the body scan meditation
- engage in drumming
- drink a hot, non-caffeinated beverage
- focus on things you find beautiful or moving
- give and receive hugs
- spend time in nature
- walk barefoot on grass or soil, immerse yourself in a body of conductive water such as the sea or a mineral-rich lake for 30 minutes at a time, as or use earthing sheets, mats, bands, or shoe straps
- do some grounding affirmations (around being present, safe, and secure) while havening
- balance your root chakra regularly
- take care of the needs of your physical body (healthy foods, hydration, sleep)

Optimizing Your Spaces Energetically

In order to keep your energy balanced, it is also important to optimize energy flow in your spaces. This is because the energy of the space you spend time in will affect you. Remember when we talked about people and how other people's energy affects our field? It is the same with spaces. In some cases, we could be dealing with good energy. If there is loving and caring atmosphere in the house, for example, the place will have a high vibrational frequency. When it is good, all we need to do is to maintain it by doing some regular space clearing. Sometimes, however, a space can have a really low vibrational frequency and needs quite a lot of clearing. This could be the case if there are frequent arguments and fights, or if there is somebody with an illness, depression, anxiety, obsessive behaviors, emotional instability, etc.

Negative energy could also be coming from objects, such as artwork, furniture, antiques, or old mirrors. If you know how to use a pendulum, you can check the energy of these kind of objects. You can also check the energy of secondhand objects you buy for your house with a pendulum. You just use the pendulum before you buy it, asking: *all things considered, is this good for me?* Also, keep in mind that energy could be lingering from previous owners. Perhaps, they had a bad relationship, or they were troubled people, or somebody was ill or died in the house. If you move into a new place, you should always do some space clearing.

If you are more sensitive, you may be picking up on the negative energy in your house, if there is any, or, indeed, any other place. This can manifest as constant fatigue, lethargy, irritation without objective reasons, insomnia, or nightmares. In fact, bad energy in your house can perpetuate any disease state. In addition, household appliances might fail, light bulbs burn out, or you may hear strange sounds and noises or pick up on strange smells. Other manifestations include plants dying (even with proper care) and animals getting sick or being constantly anxious or restless.

There are many tools you can use for space clearing. If you live in a house and you want to energetically secure the perimeter, so to speak, you can periodically sprinkle salt around your house. If you are in an apartment, you can still use salt by sprinkling it inside and leaving for a few hours before sweeping or vacuuming. Every person working with energies will tell you that salt is a superb energetic cleanser. Another thing you can do, if it is possible, is to allow only high vibration in your space. If you are in charge of where you live, if it is your house, then this will be easier to influence. But even if you live with other people, or you are unable to make these sorts of decisions, it is important that you have a little bit of your own space that you can ensure vibrates high. So, again, use salt or smudging, and keep your energy flow in check by using some of the energy hygiene strategies I shared. Make it your energetic sanctuary.

You can also diffuse essential oils to clear your spaces. The best oils for energetic cleansing include: lemongrass, eucalyptus, cypress, frankincense, oregano, orange, basil, lavender, juniper, and tea tree. Other strategies include:

- airing your spaces
- using sound (tuning forks, bells, signing bowls, chimes, drumming, signing, uplifting music)
- using gemstones such as: clear quartz, selenite, tourmaline, rose quartz, dream amethyst, orange calcite, peach selenite (most of them will need to be cleansed and charged regularly), which you can place intuitively or use specific crystal grids for specific purposes that you can look up online.

Overall, in most cases, it is easy to clear negative energy from a space. As long as you do energy clearing on a regular basis, the energy around you should be harmonious and light. That said, if you use these tools and are still picking up on strange energy, you may want to seek professional help.

Clutter

Finally, remember that clutter affects the energy of spaces. You may already know from your own experience that clutter creates overwhelm and stress. The Chinese, of course, have feng shui, an ancient practice that uses energy to harmonize individuals with their surrounding environment. The bottom line is that cluttered home is a stressful home. There are different types of clutter. Physical clutter is one type, but there are others: mental clutter, overburdened calendar, cluttered email inbox, and so on. Clutter in general increases our stress hormone levels, decreases productivity, and it overwhelms our brains, which makes us more likely to resort to coping mechanism such as comfort eating. A study from *Psychological Science* found that people who worked in a neat space where twice as likely to pick an apple to snack on vs. a chocolate bar, compared to those who worked in messy, chaotic spaces. This is why nature is so restorative. When you are near trees, ocean, or mountains, you are looking at a harmonized landscape. Clutter is a product of human activity.

So let me offer some practical strategies to de-clutter your spaces.

1. Clearing away the physical clutter: approach your house from a detached perspective, as if it is not your own house, and start with five to ten things you can remove from each room.

2. If you suffer from FOMO (fear of missing out), you need to dissect it. What is really behind your fear?

403

3. Go for less but better (quality over quantity).

4. Always ask yourself before you buy: *Do I really need this, or am I getting manipulated into buying it?*

5. Look into feng shui to further optimize your immediate environment.

Countering Geopathic Stress & EMFs

Another thing you need to do effectively in order to protect and balance your energy field is to counter the effects of geopathic stress and man-made electromagnetic fields (EMFs). Some people still poo-poo the significance of those and their impact on human health, but I promise you that this matters. Ask yourself: *If we are electromagnetic beings, how can those huge electromagnetic factors not affect us?* We are affected even by the moon cycle, after all. Collectively, geopathic stress is used to describe negative energies, which emanate from the earth and cause discomfort and ill health to those living on the surface. Earth energies can be bad, good, or neutral. Geopathic stress can be generated by ley lines, energy vortices, underground water veins, geological fissures, fault lines, and land scarring from human activity, such as railway and motorway cuttings, bridges, quarries, tunnels, mines, underground bunkers, buried gas, electricity and water mains, sewers, or building foundations.

People who have lived in the countryside have known for centuries that there are locations where livestock will get sick or die for seemingly unexplainable reasons. In 1929, Gustav von Pohl, a German scientist, got records from his local authority of people who died of cancer. He found every single one of these people lived in a place with high levels of geopathic stress. When he repeated this in other towns, he found the same. So he concluded this was a factor in their illness. This research was then repeated again with 5,300 cancer patients and the same was found. So these are really powerful energies, and buildings in these locations is inadvisable. But, of course, not many people check for that before building a house.

Issues that could be present as a result of being impacted by geopathic stress include: not feeling relaxed after a night's sleep, aching muscles and joints, emotional oversensitivity, hyperactivity or instability, headaches, anxiety, and depression. Also, the immune system will be weakened over time. These symptoms could be more or less pronounced and manifest quickly or more slowly depending on how much time the person spends close to those energy forces and how resilient they are. If somebody is sleeping on a vortex, that is bad news and will affect the body and mind sooner rather than later. We spend a lot of time sleeping, and this is where we do most of our healing, so I definitely recommend checking the areas where you sleep and spend the most time for geopathic stress.

You can check for water veins, ley lines, and vortices using dowsing. There are people who dowse remotely. There are also psychic intuitives who can connect to the place remotely and tell you how your house is doing energetically, if there are ley lines or vortices, and where. You can then re-arrange your furniture accordingly to make sure spaces where you spend most of your time in your house are free of geopathic stress. Interestingly, dogs do not like those energetic interferences, yet cats do and go towards them. So if a dog likes to go on your bed or likes to lie next to it, that space is safe, but if you have a cat that likes sleeping on your bed, it is more likely not right for you.

EMF Protection

I am only going to highlight the most important things for your consideration here. If this is an area you need to gain more knowledge in, I suggest that you follow my friend Lloyd Burrell at electricsense.com. Developing electromagnetic hypersensitivity at some point in his life put him on the path of researching this subject, which he has done now for many years. First of all, when it comes to electromagnetic radiation, it is a major stressor and it does affect everyone, although some people feel the impact more and faster than others. So if it is so detrimental to our health, why does it not affect us equally? For the same reason traumatic experiences or toxic foods do not affect everybody in the same way. It is because of the differences in the level of resilience between individuals—neurological and energetic resilience, in particular, which is what we have been building all the way through this book.

Electromagnetic hypersensitivity is also more of a problem in people with high levels of toxic metals. However, even if somebody is healthy and super resilient to begin with, if they continue being bombarded by EMFs every hour of every day, like many people are, over time, this will break them down energetically, and eventually they will experience physical symptoms. When you look at the independent research, the evidence is overwhelming that biological effects of EMFs are wide-ranging and have been linked to many different health problems, including: cancer, cardiovascular disease, diabetes, depression, premature aging, epilepsy, autism, brain tumors, infertility, insomnia, behavioral issues, tinnitus, nervous system disorders, and much more.

So we all have to be mindful of EMFs and we need to take steps to protect ourselves. Some of the key things you can do easily and right away, include:

- keep your cell phone away from you (create as much distance as possible), and if you have to have it on you, have it on flight mode

- do not bring your cell phone into your bedroom (make your bedroom an EMF-free zone)

- use a loudspeaker or headphones rather than put your phone to your head when you use it, and limit talking on your cell phone to the absolute minimum

- when you are in places with poor reception, switch your phone off, as some phones can increase their emissions 1,000-fold in areas where the signal is poor

- go wired wherever possible, rather than wireless

- use an earthing mat when you are sitting at your computer

- use protective gemstones, like black tourmaline, shungite, smokey quartz, black moonstone, or orgonites

- get some EMF-busting plants (e.g., cacti, snake plant, spider plant, stone lotus, aloe vera, asparagus fern)

- maintain good hydration levels (this goes beyond drinking water – you must have a good mineral balance)

- eat foods rich in antioxidants to counter free-radical damage and use essential oils high in antioxidants (clove, oregano, myrrh, citronella, German chamomile, coriander, fennel, cedarwood, melissa, ginger)

- supplement glutathione or boost glutathione production in the body with coffee enemas, vitamin C, selenium, turmeric, and sulphur-rich foods.

Other Tools for Biofield Optimization

To end this chapter, I want to mention some other wonderful tools I use that can help you optimize your energy field.

Bach Flower Remedies

I absolutely adore flower remedies. It is one of my favorite energy medicine modalities. They are gentle yet powerful. You may be familiar with them already, but I still encourage you to watch my video training I have provided for you in the Additional Resources. This training, accompanied with an eGuide, will teach you everything you need to know to be able to use this modality effectively.

Dowsing & Radionics

I have mentioned dowsing in passing and I want to draw your attention to it again as it is an amazing diagnostic tool. If you are interested in becoming your own health detective, check out my online program on dowsing. The extension of dowsing is radionics. Radionics is a healing technique in which our natural intuitive faculties are used both to discover the energetic disturbances underlying an illness and to encourage the return of a normal energetic field that supports health. Radionics can be used to treat not only people but animals, plants, and the soil, and can be done at a distance.

Bioresonance Technology

There is also technology that can diagnose energetic disturbances and treat them. As we said previously, the physical
body is the last body to break down when affected by a disease
process. The human body is amazing at compensating and is
always taking steps to heal. It does try to fix those energetic
disruptions for you and attempts to compensate for what is
not right. Eventually, it will not be able to do that anymore, and
you will start getting symptoms. Another reason why bioenergetics screening will show you things that you will not see on
the tests is because for most lab tests to show you a problem
you must have a considerable deterioration in function. By
then, it is more difficult to turn things around, and in some
cases, it is too late.

There are many devices on the market that can measure the
biofield, pick up on any disruptions, and then fix the problem.
This is what is called bioresonance technology, and I am a
massive fan of it. I personally have three different bioresonance
devices, two of which can be used remotely, which means I can
help people regardless of where they are in the world. If you
would like to explore this further, please contact me.

Acupuncture & Acupressure

For acupuncture you really need a practitioner who is not
only properly trained but has a good level of clinical experience addressing whatever health problem you may be dealing
with. The first time I ever went to an acupuncturist, I did not
have a good experience, which is why I am emphasizing that.
Acupressure, as you can appreciate, is not exactly the same
in terms of intensity and potential results as acupuncture, for
obvious reasons. We are talking about needles versus fingers

here. But the advantage is that you can learn to do this on yourself at home during times where it is not so easy to travel to a practitioner's office, and you can still get a lot of positive benefits. I also wanted to mention acupuncture seeds you can get and stick on your ear. That is another option if you are unable to get to an acupuncturist.

Reiki

This is another beautiful energy medicine modality. You can have in-person sessions but remember that Reiki works very well remotely, and you can also learn to do it on yourself.

I want to end this chapter by talking about interference fields, which can destabilize the autonomic nervous system. Interference fields can be a result of healed lesions, as well as concussions, root canals, or other trauma that caused stress to the body. Even though a trauma may be very old and is no longer painful, it can still interfere with the body's natural energy flow. These areas can, over time, accumulate environmental and metabolic toxins, which can cause problems and stop the body from healing. So if you have any external scars, you can begin to break up the scar tissue by manually applying shea butter, wheat germ oil, bio oil, heal gel, or diluted blue cypress essential oil for at least 30 days to address the blockage. Another thing to do is get one of those laser pointers and go over your scar drawing figures of eight, the infinity sign, along the scar. That will balance the energy flow. For internal scaring of the digestive system, digestive enzymes, taken long term, can help. You can also work with an energy healer on this.

Action points:

1. If this is not something you already do, perform a chakra assessment and use the strategies that most resonate with you to correct any imbalances you may have.

2. Decide on your daily energy hygiene routine. The more sensitive you are, the more disciplined you need to be with these procedures.

3. If you have not done this yet, take steps to declutter your spaces and make your home more EMF-free.

In Conclusion

We started this book by highlighting the true root causes of ill health and talked about how nervous system dysregulation that results from different traumas, social engineering, as well as biofield disturbances, is really at the root of most ill health. I have given you a wide range of powerful strategies, tools and techniques to rewire and rebalance your nervous system, heal your limbic system, and reprogram your subconscious mind. The key take-away here is that there are those key pillars of health: the physical factors, mind factors and energetic factors that affect each other, and there is simply no getting away from the fact that for complete healing to be possible, all these factors have to be addressed.

The physical body is the last one to break down because the body has thousands upon thousands of compensatory mechanisms but there comes a time when the body is not able to compensate any further and that is when we usually start to experience symptoms. At this point, the disease process has been in place for years, sometimes decades, but the body has been compensating, which is why you may have not been very aware of it. Once the physical body is affected, there needs to be an intervention at the physical level. We need to support the physical body and we also need to go after the true root cause, where it all started, which is the energy field and nervous system dysregulation.

But as you now know, you cannot just biohack the nervous system by using only basic vagus nerve stimulation techniques. As much as those are super helpful, they are not going to be enough on their own. There is a plethora of things that contribute to nervous system dysregulation and energetic disruptions. It is true that many of them are chemical, biological and mechanical, but the most elusive of them all are those mind and energetic factors. This is because many people are either desensitized to them or do not realize that those factors are contributing to their ill health, or how to address them. If we are going to address this nervous system dysregulation that is at the root of most chronic illness, we need to tick all the boxes highlighted in this book. This is your ultimate roadmap to healing at the psycho-energetic level.

The process of psycho-energetic healing is the same for mental or physical health issues, regardless of a label you have been assigned. When you address those pieces and bring them together into a coherent whole, you will be able to heal. Even if you have some damage at the physical level that cannot be fully repaired, this work can stop the disease process in its tracks and can certainly enhance healing beyond most people's expectations. Depending on your starting point it may take you a few weeks or a few months of doing this work to start feeling like something is shifting but the impact you can have with this work is enormous and it is certainly my opinion that this is the most worthwhile thing you can ever do for yourself. Please do remember that these emotional, mental challenges that I have been coaching you how to address in this book do come in layers. You may find that once you have worked through it once, you have experienced some shifts and then you go back to revisit certain aspects and you get more shifts. So be mindful of that.

At the beginning of this book I asked you two questions that I want to ask you again: 1) *Do you believe you are able to shape your physical health using the power of your mind?* 2) *At this moment how strongly do you believe you will be able to achieve the health you want?* How would you score your answers now, having worked through this book, on a scale of 0 to 10 (0 being nothing at all/not at all, 10 being the maximum it can be)? How do your scores compare to your initial scores? I hope that you have managed to shift along this scale. If you have made progress but would like to continue on this journey, I invite you to explore my online programs, which take you deeper into this work. I would be delighted to be able to support you going forward.

This is where I am going to end this book. I hope that this approach and materials have enhanced your life in multiple ways. I put a lot of work into creating this resource and all the feedback I have received tells me that it was worth it. I certainly enjoyed the process. I hope that going forward you will embrace what you have learned here, which means that you will be able to successfully navigate whatever life brings you from this point on. I also hope that you now trust in your own power and ability to create the exact life you have dreamed for yourself. I have a massive amount of respect for you for courageously engaging with this process and pursuing the best version of yourself. I want to wish you vibrant health, lots of joy, happiness, abundance, peace and love in your life.

Thank you for being here and letting me be part of your journey. Lots of love.

Bibliography

Ader, R. and Cohen, N. (1975). Behaviorally Conditioned Immunosuppression. Psychosom Med, vol. 37, no. 4: pp.333-340.

Andersen, S. L. and Teicher, M.H. (2012). Stress, Sensitive Periods and Maturational Events In Adolescent Depression. Trends Neurosci; 31: 183–191.

Andersen, S. L. and Teicher, M. H. (2009). Desperately driven and no brakes: developmental stress exposure and subsequent risk for substance abuse. Neurosci Biobehav Rev; Apr; 33(4):516-24.

Arnsten, A. F.T. (2000). The Biology of Being Frazzled. Science 280: 1711-1712.

Assefi, L. and Garry, M. (2003). Absolut Memory Distortions: Alcohol Placebos Influence the Misinformation Effect. Psychol Sci; vol. 14, no. 1: pp. 77-80.

Bale, T.L. (2015). Epigenetic and Transgenerational Reprogramming of Brain Development. Nat Rev Nat Sci; 16 (4), 314–319.

Baumgartner, T. et al. (2008). Oxytocin Shapes the Neural Circuitry of Trust and Trust Adaptation in Humans. Neuron; vol. 58, no. 4: pp.639-650.

Beecher, H. K. (1955). The Powerful Placebo. JAMA; vol. 159, no. 17: pp. 1602—1606.

Begley, S. and Davidson, R. (2013). The Emotional Life of Your Brain: How Its Unique Patterns Affect the Way You Think, Feel, and Live - and How You Can Change Them. Hodder Paperbacks.

Benedetti, F. et al. (1999). Inducing Placebo Respiratory Depressant Responses in Humans via Opioid Receptors. Eur J Neurosci; vol. 11, no. 2: pp.625-631.

Benedetti, F. et al. (2003). Conscious Expectation and Unconscious Conditioning in Analgesic, Motor, and Hormonal Placebo/Nocebo Responses. J Neurosci; vol. 23, no. 10: pp. 4315-4323.

Benedetti, F. et al. (2005). Neurobiological Mechanisms of the Placebo Effect. J Neurosci; vol. 25, no. 45: pp. 10390-10402.

Benson, H. (1975). The Relaxation Response. New York: Morrow.

Bradshaw, J. (1990). Home Coming: Reclaiming & Rechampioning Your Inner Child. Piatkus Books.

Brennan, B. A. (1990). Hands of Light: Guide to Healing Through the Human Energy Field: A Guide to Healing Through the Human Energy Field. Bantam Books Ltd; Reissue edition.

Bowlby, J. (1978). Attachment Theory and Its Therapeutic Implications. Adolesc Psychiatry, 6 p. 5–33.

Brown, W. A. (1998). The Placebo Effect: Should doctors be prescribing sugar pills? Sci Am 278(1): 90-95.

Burgess, T. (2011). Beliefs and How to Change Them... for Good! SRA Books.

Burgo, J. (2012). Why Do I Do That?: Psychological Defense Mechanisms and the Hidden Ways They Shape Our Lives. New Rise Press; 1st edition.

Burrell, L. (2019). EMF Practical Guide: The Simple Science of Protecting Yourself, Healing Chronic Inflammation, and Living a Naturally Healthy Life in our Toxic Electromagnetic World. AFNIL.

Cattaneo, M. G. et al. (2009). Oxytocin Stimulates in Vitro Angiogenesis via a Pyk-2/Src-Dependent Mechanism. Exp Cell Res; vol. 315, no. 18: pp. 3210-3219.

Chakravarti, A. and Little, P. (2003) Nature, Nurture and Human Disease. Nature. Jan 23; 421(6921):412-4.

Church, D. (2007). The Genie in Your Genes: Epigenetic Medicine and the New Biology of Intention. Santa Rosa, CA: Elite Books.

Cicchetti, D., Toth, S. L. and Hennessy, K. (1989). Research on the Consequences of Child Maltreatment and Its Application to Educational Settings. Topics in Early Childhood Spec Educ; 9(2), 33-55.

Cohen, J. A. et al. (2002). Treating Traumatized Children: Clinical Implications of the Psychobiology of Posttraumatic Stress Disorder. Trauma, Violence, & Abuse; 3(2), 91-108.

Cohen, P. (2001). Mental Gymnastics Increase Bicep Strength. New Scientist; vol. 172, no. 2318: p. 17.

Cole, P. M. and Putnam, F. W. (1992). Effect of Incest on Self and Social Functioning: A Developmental Psychopathology Perspective. J Consult Clin Psychol; 60(2), 174.

Cousins, N. (1976). Anatomy of an Illness (as Perceived by the Patient). N Engl J Med; vol. 295, no. 26: pp. 1458—1463.

Crum, A. J. and Langer, E. J. (2007). Mind-Set Matters: Exercise and the Placebo Effect, Psychol Sci; vol. 18, no. 2: pp. 165—171.

Dale, C. (2013). The Subtle Body Practice Manual: A Comprehensive Guide to Energy Healing. Sounds True Inc; illustrated edition.

Dana, D. (2020). Polyvagal Exercises for Safety and Connection: 50 Client-Centered Practices (Norton Series on Interpersonal Neurobiology). W. W. Norton & Company.

Dar-Nimrod, I. and Heine, S. J. (2006). Exposure to Scientific Theories Affects Women's Math Performance. Science; vol. 314, no. 5798:p. 435.

Davidson, R. J., Jackson, D. C. and Kalin, N. H. (2000). Emotion, Plasticity, Context, and Regulation: Perspectives from Affective Neuroscience. Psychol Bullletin, 126(6), 890.

De Bellis, M. D. et al. (1999). Developmental Traumatology Part I: Biological Stress Systems. Biol Psych; 45(10), 1259-1270.

De Bellis, M. D. et al. (1999). Developmental Traumatology Part II: Brain Development. Biol Psych; 45(10), 1271-1284.

De la Fuente-Fernândez, R. T. et al. (2001). Expectation and Dopamine Release: Mechanism of the Placebo Effect in Parkinson's Disease. Science; vol. 293, no. 5532: pp. 1164—1166.

Desharnais, R. et al. (1993). Aerobic Exercise and the Placebo Effect: A Controlled Study. Psych Med; vol. 55, no. 2: pp. 149-154.

Dillon, K. M., Minchoff, B. and Baker, K. H. (1985-1986) Positive Emotional States and Enhancement of the Immune System. Int J Psych Med; vol. 15, no. 1: pp. 13-18.

Discovery (2003). Placebo: Mind Over Medicine? Medical Mysteries. Silver Spring, MD, Discovery Health Channel.

Dispenza, J. (2012). Breaking the Habit of Being Yourself: How to Lose Your Mind and Create a New One. Hay House UK.

Dispenza, J. (2014). You Are the Placebo: Making Your Mind Matter, Hay House UK.

Dodic, M. et al. (2002). Programming Effects of Short Prenatal Exposure to Cortisol. Fed Am Soc Exp Biol; 16: 1017-1026.

Dodge, K. A. and Price, J. M. (1994). On the Relation between Social Information Processing and Socially Competent Behavior in Early School-aged Children. Child Develop; 65(5), 1385-1397.

Dube S.R. et al. (2009). Cumulative Childhood Stress and Autoimmune Diseases in Adults. Psych Med; 71(2): 243-250.

Erickson, M. F. and Egeland, B. (2002). Child Neglect. The APSAC Handbook on Child Maltreatment, 2, 3-20.

Fehmiand L. and Robbins J. (2007). The Open-Focus Brain: Harnessing the Power of Attention to Heal Mind and Body. Boston: Trumpeter Books.

Felitti, V.J. et al. (1998). Relationship of Childhood Abuse and Household Dysfunction to Many of the Leading Causes of Death in Adults: the Adverse Childhood Experiences (ACE) Study. Am J Prev Med; 1998; 14, 245–258.

Fraga, M. F. et al. (2005). Epigenetic Differences Arise During the Lifetime of Monozygotic Twins. Proc Natl Acad Sci USA; vol. 102, no. 30: pp.10604-10609.

Fransson, E. et al. (2012). Negative Emotions and Cytokines in Maternal and Cord Serum at Preterm Birth. Am J Reprod Immunol; Jun;67 (6):506-14.

Geers, L. et al. (2007). Further Evidence for Individual Differences in Placebo Responding: An Interactionist Perspective. J Psych Res; vol. 62, no. 5: pp.563-570.

Gerber, R. (2001). A Practical Guide to Vibrational Medicine: Energy Healing and Spiritual Transformation. William Morrow Paperbacks.

Gluckman, P. D. and Hanson, M. A. (2004). Living with the Past: Evolution, Development, and Patterns of Disease. Science 305: 1733-1736.

Goldstein, L. E. et al. (1996). Role of the Amygdala in the Coordination of Behavioral, Neuroendocrine, and Prefrontal Cortical Monoamine Responses to Psychological Stress in the Rat. J Neurosci; 16(15): 4787-4798.

Greenberg, G. (2003). Is It Prozac? Or Placebo? Mother Jones: 76-81.

Greenblatt, J.M. and Dimino, J. (2016). Evidence-Based Research on the Role of Zinc and Magnesium Deficiencies in Depression. Psych Times; Dec.

Grinder, J. and Bandler, R. (1976) The Structure of Magic. Science and Behavior Books, Inc.

Guillot, A. et al. (2007). Muscular Responses During Motor Imagery as a Function of Muscle Contraction Types. Int J Psych; vol. 66, no. 1: pp. 18-27.

Habib, N. (2019). Activate Your Vagus Nerve: Unleash Your Body's Natural Ability to Heal. Ulysses Press; Illustrated edition.

Hamilton, D. R. (2010). How Your Mind Can Heal Your Body. Carlsbad, CA: Hay House.

Harris, T. A. (1973). I'm OK – You're OK. Pan Books Ltd.

Hart, J., Gunnar, M. and Cicchetti, D. (1996). Altered Neuroendocrine Activity in Maltreated Children Related to Symptoms of Depression. Dev Psychopathol; 8(1), 201-214.

Hawkins, D. R. (2015). Transcending the Levels of Consciousness: The Stairway to Enlightenment Hay House UK; Reprint edition.

Hay, L. (1984). You Can Heal Your Life Hay House; New edition.

Hayashi, T. et al. (2007). Laughter Up-Regulates the Genes Related to NK Cell Activity in Diabetes. Biomed Res (Tokyo, Japan), vol. 28, no. 6: pp. 281—285.

Heim, C. and Nemeroff, C. B. (2009). Neurobiology of Posttraumatic Stress Disorder. CNS spectr, 14(1 suppl. 1), 13-24.

Heim, C. and Nemeroff, C. (2001). The Role of Childhood Trauma in the Neurobiology of Mood and Anxiety Disorders: Preclinical and Clinical Studies. Biol Psych; June 49(12): 1023-1039.

Heller, L. and Lapierre, A. (2012). Healing Developmental Trauma: How Early Trauma Affects Self-Regulation, Self-Image, and the Capacity for Relationship. North Atlantic Books, U.S.

Hickok, et al. (2001). The Role of Patients' Expectations in the Development of Anticipatory

House, D.E. (1993). Evidence for Direct Effect of Magnetic Fields on Neurite Outgrowth. FASEB Journal, vol. 7, no. 9: pp. 801-806.

Holden, C. (1996).Child Development: Small Refugees Suffer the Effects of Early Neglect. Science 274(5290): 1076-1077.

Holden, C. (2003). Future Brightening for Depression Treatments. Science 302: 810-813.

Horgan, J. (1999). Chapter 4: Prozac and Other Placebos. The Undiscovered Mind: How the Human Brain Defies Replication, Medication, and Explanation. New York, The Free Press: 102-136.

Ikemi, Y. and Nakagawa, S. (1962). A Psychosomatic Study of Contagious Dermatitis. Kyushu J Med Sci; vol. 13: pp. 335—350.

Jackman, R. (2020). Healing Your Lost Inner Child: How to Stop Impulsive Reactions, Set Healthy Boundaries and Embrace an Authentic Life. Practical Wisdom Press.

Jacobs Hendel, H. (2018). It's Not Always Depression: Working the Change Triangle to Listen to the Body, Discover Core Emotions, and Connect to Your Authentic Self. Penguin Life.

Jung, Y. et al. (2019). Relationships Among Stress, Emotional Intelligence, Cognitive Intelligence, and Cytokines. Observ Study Med; May; 98(18):e15345.

Kajeepeta, S. et al. (2015). Adverse Childhood Experiences Are Associated With Adult Sleep Disorders: a Systematic Review. Sleep Med; 16(3):320-330.

Kaptchuk, T. J. et al. (2010). Placebos Without Deception: A Randomized Controlled Trial in Irritable Bowel Syndrome. PLOS ONE, vol. 5, no. 12: p. el 5591.

Kiecolt-Glaser, J. K. et al. (2002). Emotions, Morbidity, and Mortality: New Perspectives from Psychoneuroimmunology. Annu Rev Psychol; 53:83-107.

Kim, S. et al. (2017). Visualizing the Neurobiology of Trauma: Design and Evaluation of an eLearning Module for Continuing Professional Development of Family Physicians in the Online Psychiatric Education Network. J Biocom; 41(2).

Kirkley, A. et al. (2008). Randomized Trial of Arthroscopic Surgery for Osteoarthritis of the Knee. N Engl J Med; vol. 359, no. 11: pp. 1097-1107.

Kirsch I. et al. (2002). The Emperor's New Drugs: An Analysis of Antidepressants Medication Data Submitted to the U.S. Food and Drug Administration. Prevention & Treatment (American Psychological Association) 5: Article 23.

Kirsch, I. and Sapirstein, G. (1998). Listening to Prozac but Hearing Placebo: A Meta-analysis of Antidepressant Medication. Prevent Treat; vol. 1, no. 2: article 00002a.

Kirsch, I. et al. (2008). Initial Severity and Antidepressant Benefits: A Meta-analysis of Data Submitted to the Food and Drug Administration. PLOS Med; vol. 5, no.2: p. e45.

Klopfer, B. (1957). Psychological Variables in Human Cancer. J Prot Tech; vol. 21, no. 4: pp. 331—340.

Kok, B. E. et al. (2013). How Positive Emotions Build Physical Health: Perceived Positive Social Connections Account for the Upward Spiral Between Positive Emotions and Vagal Tone. Psychol Sci; vol. 24, no. 7:pp. 1123-1132.

Kopp, M. S. and Réthelyi, J. (2004). Where Psychology Meets Physiology: Chronic Stress and Premature Mortality—The Central-Eastern European Health Paradox. Brain Res Bull; vol. 62, no. 5: pp. 351—367.

Leuchter, A. F. et al. (2002). Changes in Brain Function of Depressed Subjects during Treatment with Placebo. Am J Psych; vol. 159, no. 1: pp. 122—129.

Leutwyler, K. (1998). Don't Stress: It is Now Known to Cause Developmental Problems, Weight Gain and Neurodegeneration. Sci Am; 28-30.

Lesage, J. et al. (2004). Prenatal Stress Induces Intrauterine Growth Restriction and Programmes Glucose Intolerance and Feeding Behaviour Disturbances in the Aged Rat. J Endocrinol; 181: 291-296.

Levine, A. and Heller, R. (2019). Attached: Are you Anxious, Avoidant or Secure? How the science of adult attachment can help you find – and keep – love Bluebird; Main Market edition.

Levine, J. D., Gordon, N. C. and Fields, H. L. (1978). The Mechanism of Placebo Analgesia. Lancet, vol. 2, no. 8091: pp. 654—657.

Levine, P. (1997). Waking The Tiger: Healing Trauma. North Atlantic Books, Berkeley CA.

Levy, B. R. et al. (2002). Longevity Increased by Positive Self-perceptions of Aging. J Person Soc Psychol; vol. 83, no. 2: pp. 261—270.

Lewis, D. O. et al. (1986). Psychiatric, Neurological, and Psychoeducational Characteristics of 15 Death Row Inmates in the United States. Am J Psych; 143(7), 838-845.

Lipton, B. (2005). The Biology of Belief. Unleashing the Power of Consciousness, Matter & Miracles. Hay House Inc.

Luparello, T. et al. (1968). Influences of Suggestion on Airway Reactivity in Asthmatic Subjects. Psych Med; vol. 30, no. 6: pp. 819—829.

Ma'ati Smith, J. (2013). The Chakras for Beginners: Essential Aura and Chakra Balancing for Wellness. CreateSpace Independent Publishing Platform.

Madison, T. (2019). Enneagram: #1 Made Easy Guide to the 9 Type of Personalities. Grow Your Self-Awareness, Evolve Your Personality, and build Healthy Relationships. Create Your Reality.

Maruta, T. et al. (2002). Optimism-Pessimism Assessed in the 1960s and Self-Reported Health Status 30 Years Later. Mayo Clinic Proceedings, vol. 77, no. 8: pp.748-753.

Mason, A. A. (1952). A Case of Congenital Ichthyosiform Erythrodermia of Brocq Treated by Hypnosis. Brit Med J; 30: 442-443.

Meyers, B. A. (2013). Pemf - the Fifth Element of Health: Learn Why Pulsed Electromagnetic Field (Pemf) Therapy Supercharges Your Health Like Nothing Else! BalboaPress; Illustrated edition.

McClare, C. W. (1974). Resonance in Bioenergetics. Ann N Y Acad Sci; vol. 227: 74-97.

McEwen, B. S. and Seeman, T. (1999). Protective and Damaging Effects of Mediators of Stress. Elaborating and Testing the Concepts of Allostasis and Allostatic Load. Ann N Y Acad Sci; vol. 896: pp.30-47.

McLaren, K. (2010). The Language of Emotions: What Your Feelings Are Trying to Tell You. Sounds True Inc.

Moseley, J. B. et al. (2002). A Controlled Trial of Arthroscopic Surgery for Osteoarthritis of the Knee. N Engl J Med; 347(2): 81-88.

Myss, C. (1997). Anatomy Of The Spirit: The Seven Stages of Power and Healing. Bantam.

Myss, C. (1998). Why People Don't Heal And How They Can: a guide to healing and overcoming physical and mental illness. Bantam; 1st Paperback.

Nathanielsz, P. W. (1999). Life In the Womb: The Origin of Health and Disease. Ithaca, NY, Promethean Press.

Newbigging, S. C. (2019) Mind Detox: Discover and Resolve the Root Causes of Chronic Conditions and Persistent Problems. Findhorn Press; 2nd edition.

Northrup, C. (2019). Dodging Energy Vampires: An Empath's Guide to Evading Relationships That Drain You and Restoring Your Health and Power Hay House Inc; Reprint edition.

Odoul, M. (2018). What Your Aches and Pains Are Telling You: Cries of the Body, Messages from the Soul Healing Arts Press; Illustrated edition.

Orloff, J. (2019). Thriving as an Empath: 365 Days of Self-Care for Sensitive People Sounds True Inc.

Opendak, M. and Sullivan, R.M. (2016) Unique Neurobiology During The Sensitive Period For Attachment Produces Distinctive Infant Trauma Processing. Eur J Psychotraumatol; 7:10.3402.

Oschman, J. L. (2006). Trauma Energetics. J Bodyw Mov Ther; vol. 10, no. 1: pp. 21—34.

Paul, M. (1990). Healing Your Aloneness: Finding Love and Wholeness Through Your Inner Child. Bravo Ltd; 1st edition.

Paus, T., Keshavan, M. and Giedd, J.N. (2008). Why Do Many Psychiatric Disorders Emerge During Adolescence? Nat Rev Neurosci; 9(12): 947–57.

Pert, C.B. (1997). Molecules of Emotion. Why You Feel the Way You Feel. Scribner, New York.

Pesonen, A.K. et al. (2010). Childhood Separation Experience Predicts HPA Axis Hormonal Responses in Late Adulthood: A Natural Experiment of World War II. Psychoneuroendocrinology; 35(5):758-767.

Pitman, R. K. (1989). Post-traumatic Stress Disorder, Hormones, and Memory. Biol Psych; 26(3), 221-223.

Poole Heller, D. (2019). The Power of Attachment: How to Create Deep and Lasting Intimate Relationships Sounds True Inc.

Popp, F.A. (1998). Biophotons and Their Regulatory Role in Cells. Frontier Perspectives, vol. 7, no. 2: pp. 13-22.

Porges, S. W. (2021). Polyvagal Safety: Attachment, Communication, Self-Regulation. W.W. Norton & Co.

Pribram, K. H. (2013). The Form Within: My Point of View. Prospecta Press.

Radin, D. (2009). The Noetic Universe. The Scientific Evidence for Psychic Phenomena. Transworld Publishers, London.

Raghupathi, W. and Raghupathi, V. (2018). An Empirical Study of Chronic Diseases in the United States: A Visual Analytics Approach to Public Health. Int J Environ Res Public Health; Mar; 15(3): 431.

Ranganathan, V. K. et al. (2004). From Mental Power to Muscle Power: Gaining Strength by Using the Mind. Neuropsychologia; vol. 42, no. 7: pp. 944-956.

Rankin, L. (2020). Mind Over Medicine: Scientific Proof That You Can Heal Yourself Hay House Inc; revised edition.

Rauch, S. L. et al. (1996). A Symptom Provocation Study of Posttraumatic Stress Disorder Using Positron Emission Tomography and Script-driven Imagery. Arch Gen Psych; 53(5), 380-387.

Reeves, R. R. et al. (2007). Nocebo Effects with Antidepressant Clinical Drug Trial Placebos. Gen Hosp Psych; vol. 29, no. 3: pp. 275—277.

Robertson, I. (2000). Mind Sculpture: Unlocking Your Brain's Untapped Potential. New York: Bantam Books.

Rosenzweig, M. R. and Bennett, E. L. (1996). Psychobiology of Plasticity: Effects of Training and Experience on Brain and Behavior. Behav Brain Res; vol. 78, no. 1: pp. 57—65.

Rossi, E. L. (2002). The Psychobiology of Gene Expression: Neuroscience and Neurogenesis in Hypnosis and the Healing Arts. New York: W. W. Norton and Company.

Rossi, E.L. (1994). The Psychobiology of Mind-Body Healing. New Concepts of Therapeutic Hypnosis. W.W. Norton & Co., New York.

Roy, S. et al. (2005). Wound Site Neutrophil Transcriptome in Response to Psychological Stress in Young Men. Gene Expression; vol. 12, no. 4—6: pp. 273—287.

Rozee, P. D. and van Boemel, G. (1989). The Psychological Effects of War Trauma and Abuse on Older Cambodian Refugee Women. Women and Therapy; vol. 8, no. 4: pp. 23-50.

Ruden, R. A. (2010) When the Past Is Always Present: Emotional Traumatization, Causes, and Cures. Routledge; 1st edition.

Ruden, R. A. (2017). Havening Techniques®: A Primer. Ronald A. Ruden.

Rusk, T. and Read, R. (1986). I Want to Change But I Don't Know How. Price/Stern/Sloan Publishers, Inc., Los Angeles.

Ryle, G. (1949). The Concept of Mind. Chicago, University of Chicago Press.

Sandman, C. A. et al. (1994). Psychobiological Influences of Stress and HPA Regulation on the Human Fetus and Infant Birth Outcomes. Ann N Y Acad Sci; 739 (Models of Neuropeptide Action): 198-210.

Sareen, J. (2014). Posttraumatic Stress Disorder in Adults: Impact, Comorbidity, Risk Factors, and Treatment. Can J Psych; 59(9), 460-467.

Schauer, M. and Elbert, T. (2010). Dissociation Following Traumatic Stress: Etiology and Treatment. J Psychol; 218(2), 109-127.

Schore, J. R. and Schore, A. N. (2008). Modern Attachment Theory: The Central Role of Affect Regulation in Development and Treatment. Clin Soc Work J; 36(1), 9-20.

Schuler, L.A., Auger, A.P. (2010). Psychosocially Influenced Cancer: Diverse Early-Life Stress Experiences and Links to Breast Cancer. Cancer prevention research (Philadelphia, Pa); 3(11):1365-1370.

Scott-Mumby, K. (2015). Medicine Beyond: New Dimensions of Biology and Healing Beyond the Everyday Laws of Physics. Supernoetics, Inc.

Segerstrom, S. C. and Miller, G. E. (2004). Psychological Stress and the Human Immune System: A Meta-analytic Study of 30 Years of Inquiry. Psychol Bull; vol. 130, no. 4: pp. 601—630.

Sherin, J. E. and Nemeroff, C. B. (2011). Post-traumatic Stress Disorder: the Neurobiological Impact of Psychological Trauma. Dial Clin Neurosci; 13(3), 263.

Siegel, D. J. (1999). The Developing Mind: How Relationships and the Brain Interact to Shape Who We Are. New York, Guilford.

Siegel, D. J. (2007). The Mindful Brain: Reflection and Attunement in the Cultivation of Well-Being. New York: W. W. Norton and Company.

Smyth, N. et al. (2015). Anxious Attachment Style Predicts an Enhanced Cortisol Response to Group Psychosocial Stress. Int J Biol Stress; 18(2).

Solomon, E.P., Heide, K. (2005). The Biology of Trauma: Implications for Treatment. J Interpers Violence; 20(1):51-60.

Springer, K.W. et al. (2003). The Long-term Health Outcomes of Childhood Abuse: An Overview and a Call to Action. J Gen Intern Med; 18(10):864-870.

Stanton, M. E., Gutierrez, Y. R., and Levine, S. (1988). Maternal Deprivation Potentiates Pituitary-adrenal Stress Responses in Infant Rats. Behav Neurosci; 102(5), 692.

Szalavitz, M. and Perry, B. (2010). Born For Love. William Morrow.

Tiller, J. (2015). I love... Affirmations for a Life Worth Living. Amazon Publishing.

Tugade, M. M. and Fredrickson, B. L. (2004). Resilient Individuals Use Positive Emotions to Bounce Back from Negative Emotional Experiences. J Pers Soc Psychol; Feb: 86(2):320-33.

Tugade, M. M. et al. (2004). Psychological Resilience and Positive Emotional Granularity: Examining the Benefits of Positive Emotions on Coping and Health. J Pers; Dec: 72(6):1161-90.

Van der Kolk, B.A. (2014). The Body Keeps the Score: Mind, Brain and Body in the Transformation of Trauma. Penguin; 1st edition.

Van der Kolk, B. A. (2003). The Neurobiology of Childhood Trauma and Abuse. Child Adolesc Psych Clin N Am; 12(2), 293-318.

Van der Kolk, B.A. et al. (2005). Disorders of Extreme Stress: the Empirical Foundation of a Complex Adaptation to Trauma. J Trauma Stress; Oct 2005; 18(5): 388-99.

Van der Kolk, B. A. and Fisler, R. E. (1994). Childhood Abuse and Neglect and Loss of Self-regulation. Bulll Menninger Clin; 58(2), 145.

Walsh, B. T. et al. (2002). Placebo Response in Studies of Major Depression: Variable, Substantial, and Growing. JAMA. 2002; 287(14):1840-1847.

Walsh, W.J., Glab, L.B. and Haakenson, M.L. (2004). Reduced Violent Behavior Following Biochemical Therapy. Physiol Behav; Oct; 82(5): 835-9.

Webb, J. (2019). Running on Empty: Overcome Your Childhood Emotional Neglect. Morgan James Publishing.

Wiener, S. G., Lowe, E. L., and Levine, S. (1992). Pituitary-adrenal Response to Weaning in Infant Squirrel Monkeys. Psychobiology, 20(1), 65-70.

White, J. and Krippner, S. (1977). Future Science: Life Energies and the Physics of Paranormal Phenomena Mass Market Paperback. Anchor Books; 1st edition.

Yue, G. and Cole, K. J. (1992). Strength Increases from the Motor Program: Comparison of Training with Maximal Voluntary and

Imagined Muscle Contractions. J Neurophysiol; vol. 67, no. 5:pp. 1114-1123.

Zellik, N. et al. (2004). Range of Neurologic Disorders in Patients with Celiac Disease. Pediatrics; June 2004; 113(6):1672-6.